Sports Medicine

For Young Athletes

Sports Medicine

For Young Athletes

A Guide for Parents, Teachers, and Coaches

By the Institute for Athletic Medicine
Edited by Scott Kulstad, MEd, ATC/R

Fairview Press
Minneapolis

Published by Fairview Press
2450 Riverside Avenue South
Minneapolis, MN 55454.

Library of Congress Cataloging-in-Publication Data

Sports Medicine for Young Athletes / by the Institute for Athletic Medicine; edited by Scott Kulstad

p. cm.
Includes bibliographical references and index.
ISBN 1-57749-066-5 (alk. paper)
1. Sports medicine—Popular works. I. Kulstad, Scott.
II. Institute for Athletic Medicine.
RC1210.P27 1998
617.1'027—dc21 98-16095
CIP

First Printing: August 1998

Printed in the United States of America
02 01 00 99 98 7 6 5 4 3 2 1

Cover design: Laurie Duren
Interior design: Percolator Graphic Design

Contents

Preface

Parents are dedicated folks. They drive their sons and daughters to practices, sometimes even coaching sports about which they know very little. Parents do this because of their love and concern for their children. We applaud this.

We also applaud youth sport programs. From youth soccer to high-school wrestling, we firmly believe that athletic activities are great for people of all ages. When we say athletics, we do not mean only organized sports. Recreational play is a great way for children—and adults—to improve physical fitness and overall health.

Yet, with physical activity sometimes comes injury. We have all heard the comment, "Nothing is sure in life, except death and taxes." We could add to this, saying, "Nothing is sure in life, except death, taxes, and injury (at some point) if you are active." People get hurt—no matter how young or old they are—especially when they are active. That is the reason for this book.

We know that coaches and parents of athletic youngsters have a tremendous responsibility. Caring for the physical welfare of children is a stressful job—especially if sports medicine seems foreign. To many people, sports medicine is as foreign as car repair is to me! We want this book to help you take care of your child or player.

The purpose of this book, then, is twofold: to educate and to empower. We hope that we can educate the uninformed by making anatomy and sports medicine understandable. For that reason, we have tried to limit the number of complicated terms we use. We have attempted to explain things with logical analogies and easy-to-understand definitions, and we have provided illustrations of the major bones, muscles, and tendons discussed throughout this book.

We want to empower you as well. As much as some people may wish for others to bear the responsibility for their children's healthcare, today's healthcare climate may not allow that luxury. Managed-care companies may dictate when and from whom you seek medical attention for your child's injuries. Your ability to determine when a child needs emergency care and when you can treat the problem at home will ultimately save you time and energy. While emergency room and urgent care physicians are very knowledgeable, many do not understand sports medicine the way an orthopedist or a family physician may. We should not expect that emergency room personnel will know everything about sports medicine—just as we wouldn't expect an orthopedic surgeon to have expertise in advanced life support or emergency medicine. Therefore, depending on the ailment, you may get better care by waiting. Later chapters include information about those times when you may want to wait and schedule an appointment with your doctor. We also discuss when you cannot afford to wait.

In organizing this book, we have put "first things first," to quote famous author Stephen Covey, by first discussing anatomy and physiology. We review the different systems in the body and discuss how each system relates to sports medicine. For example, when we discuss the skin, we highlight its function and also identify certain skin infections. Parents of wrestlers will certainly benefit from this. When we discuss the cardiovascular system, we mention possible causes for faintness and breathing difficulties that an athlete may experience. The anatomy chapter also discusses how the body responds to injury, answering common questions like, "Why does my son's ankle swell when he sprains it?" Finally, we include diagrams of the major bone and muscle groups on pages 4 through 7.

The chapter on exercise and conditioning discusses what young children can do to strengthen their bodies and how they can stay in shape. We do not expect you to walk away from this chapter with the answer to every strength and conditioning question. However, we do hope that it satisfies an interest and raises specific questions you may have for your physician or an athletic trainer. Athletic trainer Jim Rakow answers the most common questions parents ask.

We devote an entire chapter to injury evaluation, treatment, and prevention. Although it is impossible to prevent all injuries, this chapter should help you find ways to prevent many common injuries. Even without the skills of a physician, physical therapist, or athletic trainer, you can learn how to look at an injury knowledgeably. Too often, the prospect of injury scares parents, and the thought of locating the problem is simply overwhelming. This chapter will teach you how to evaluate an injury objectively and respond accordingly. Two athletic trainers with an incredible amount of experience wrote this chapter. One served as the athletic trainer for the Gold Medal 1980 U.S. Olympic hockey team, and the other earned a Distinguished Achievement Award from the National Athletic Trainer's Association. Their biographies are included at the end of the chapter.

An important chapter in this book is the chapter on emergency procedures. Effectively managing the treatment of an injury may be the greatest service you can provide for your child or the player in your charge. Failing to properly manage injuries places you at risk, and may put the athlete in harm's way. Red flag icons ( ) alert you to signs and symptoms to which you should give special attention. Some may instruct you to seek emergency care, while others may suggest another course of action.

All parents and coaches should read the chapter titled Issues for Girls and Women Only. This chapter is dedicated to the issues concerning female athletes. Did you know that many adolescent women suffer from incontinence, especially if they participate in sports like cross-country and track? Moreover, many young women are too embarrassed to discuss this with their parents or health-care provider. Keeping the issue a secret prolongs the problem. Our physical therapists, who have received special training in this issue, discuss stress incontinence and provide ideas for treatment. The authors discuss other issues as well, including anorexia (a life-threatening illness), osteoporosis, and amenorrhea.

The chapters in Part Two of this book address injuries specific to certain body parts. For quick reference about a knee injury, you may refer directly to the chapter on knees. You may find some overlapping information from one chapter to the next, but this is intentional. Some people may wish to read about knee injuries, for example. Others may wish to read about thigh injuries. In reality, however, the muscles that act on the knee originate in the thigh.

Within these subject-specific chapters, we offer simple, straightforward answers to frequently asked questions like, "How do I know if it's broken?" While our answers may sound similar from one chapter to the next, keep in mind that this is designed to be a quick reference section. One section will not build upon another.

Acknowledgments

To my wife, Hayley, and my son, Alex, I thank you for your support while I worked on this book. I love you dearly. Hayley and Alex spent several days and nights upstairs while I was downstairs typing. I greatly appreciate their patience, and this book is much better because of their continued support. On behalf of our contributing authors, I am sure they also thank their families. Many people invested time and energy into this book. Their families deserve thanks as well.

To Fairview Press editors Jessica Thoreson, Lori Coleman, and Stephanie Billecke goes tremendous gratitude. Their comments and suggestions have made this book much better. Without them, we would still be writing, and you would likely never understand the final product.

To Jim Rakow, you deserve as much credit as anybody for the success of this book. From the very beginning, you encouraged and helped. With all sincerity, thank you.

To my student-athletes at Orono High School, who volunteered as models and encouraged this book from the beginning, I owe appreciation. Erin Albers, Erin Shaughnessy, Amy Gillum, Kami Jellison, and Graig Gorder (and many more) are students who underscore my belief that tomorrow's America is in great hands. These students have restored my faith that our young adults are caring and compassionate people. They are also dedicated and driven for success, on and off the athletic field. I will truly celebrate the day when their contributions empower and influence more than just the few people who surround them daily.

To Steve Fedie, Orono High School Athletic Director, thank you for fostering an athletic program that encourages and uplifts young people. Thank you for making the services of an athletic trainer available to your coaches, student-athletes, and their parents. Most importantly, thank you for allowing me to serve as your athletic trainer for five wonderful years.

To the Institute for Athletic Medicine administration, who supported this project even during its most difficult times, thank you. Sue Lewis, I hope you enjoy this book and like the final product. We do.

Finally, we owe you, the parents and coaches, a debt of gratitude. Your dedication to this book demonstrates a dedication and concern for your children and your players. We are sincerely grateful to you for allowing us to help. Thank you for allowing us into your games and your practices, and thank you for letting us teach you. Thank you for being empowered and for learning. Your children and players will benefit greatly!

Scott Kulstad, MEd, ATC/R
Editor and Contributing Author

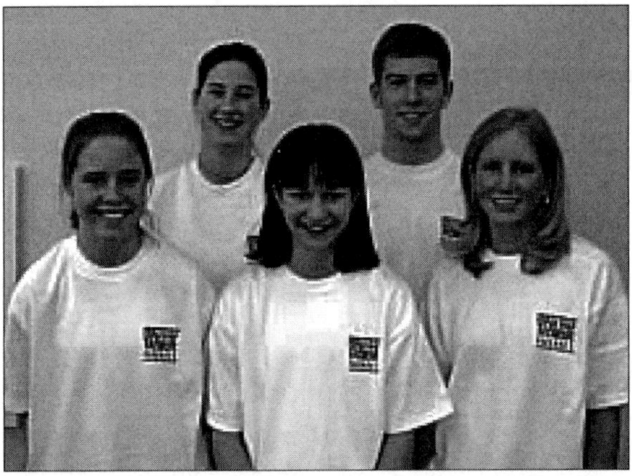

The students you see here are high-school athletes. One will play college football. One plays on an Olympic Development volleyball team. Three others play soccer. They all have one thing in common—they have suffered sports-related injuries. Every one of them, however, has fully recuperated from his or her injuries and remains active. Like these kids, your children will get hurt, and they will recover.

Part One:

The Basics

Chapter 1

Anatomy and Physiology

Have you ever looked at a picture of a skeleton, or a diagram of the muscles and organs in the human body? Chances are, you have seen a chart like this on the wall at a doctor's office. However, you probably can't remember all the details of how everything fits together.

Here's a good chance for you to "bone up" on your knowledge of anatomy (the structures of the body) and physiology (how these structures work). When you have a basic understanding of the systems of the body, you are helping yourself, your family, and your healthcare provider. Educated athletes, parents, and coaches can more easily identify injuries in themselves and in the young people in their care if they understand the basics. In addition, you can help make sure that an injured person gets proper treatment if you can clearly explain a problem to a doctor or emergency medical technician. "My daughter has pain over her lateral collateral ligament" gives a medical professional a lot more information than "my daughter's arm hurts." When you know a few facts about how the systems work together in a healthy body, you may understand why a medical professional recommends one form of treatment or exercise instead of another.

This chapter gives you a basic overview of systems that aren't discussed elsewhere in this book. If you want to learn more about anatomy and physiology, a medical professional can direct you to helpful sources.

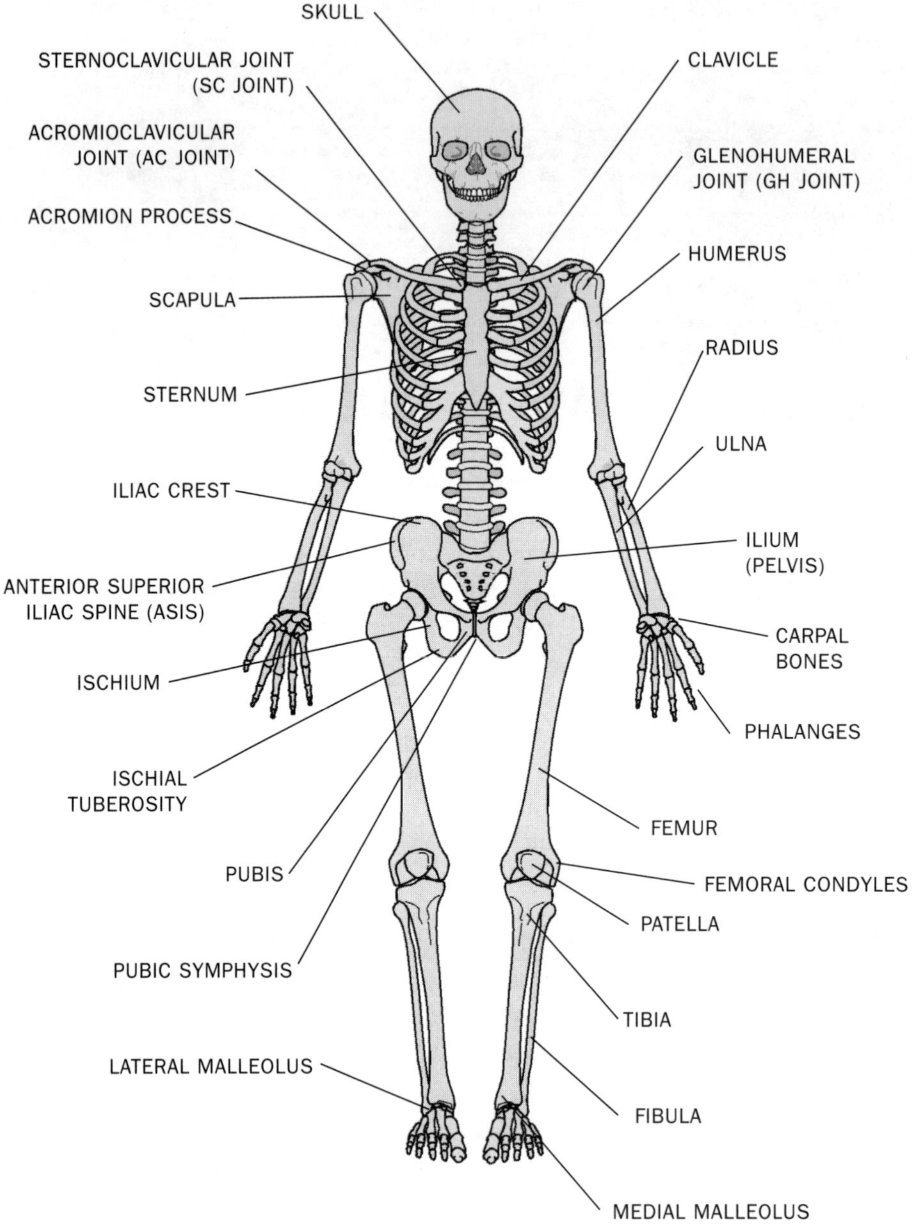
SKULL
STERNOCLAVICULAR JOINT (SC JOINT)
CLAVICLE
ACROMIOCLAVICULAR JOINT (AC JOINT)
GLENOHUMERAL JOINT (GH JOINT)
ACROMION PROCESS
HUMERUS
SCAPULA
RADIUS
STERNUM
ULNA
ILIAC CREST
ILIUM (PELVIS)
ANTERIOR SUPERIOR ILIAC SPINE (ASIS)
CARPAL BONES
ISCHIUM
PHALANGES
ISCHIAL TUBEROSITY
FEMUR
PUBIS
FEMORAL CONDYLES
PATELLA
PUBIC SYMPHYSIS
TIBIA
LATERAL MALLEOLUS
FIBULA
MEDIAL MALLEOLUS

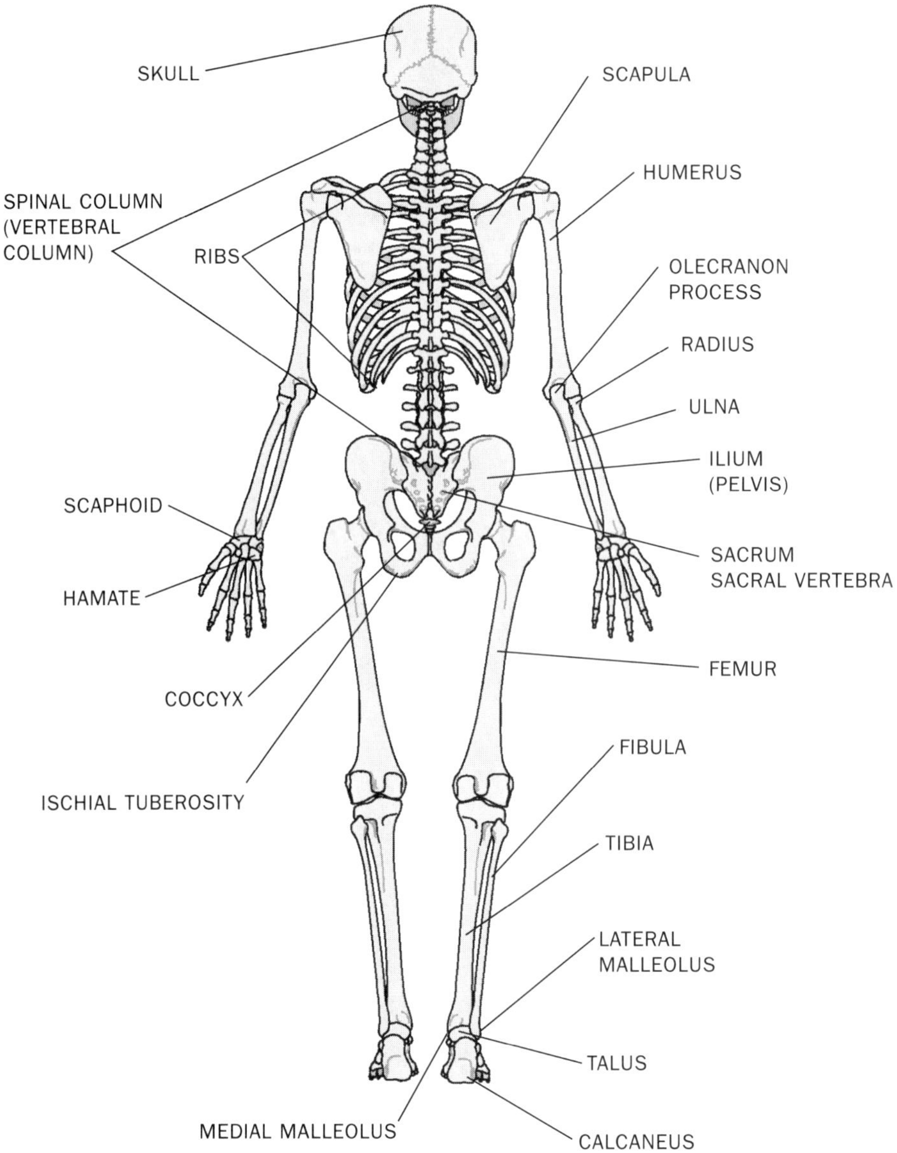
SKULL
SCAPULA
HUMERUS
SPINAL COLUMN
(VERTEBRAL
COLUMN)
RIBS
OLECRANON
PROCESS
RADIUS
ULNA
ILIUM
(PELVIS)
SCAPHOID
SACRUM
SACRAL VERTEBRA
HAMATE
FEMUR
COCCYX
FIBULA
ISCHIAL TUBEROSITY
TIBIA
LATERAL
MALLEOLUS
TALUS
MEDIAL MALLEOLUS
CALCANEUS

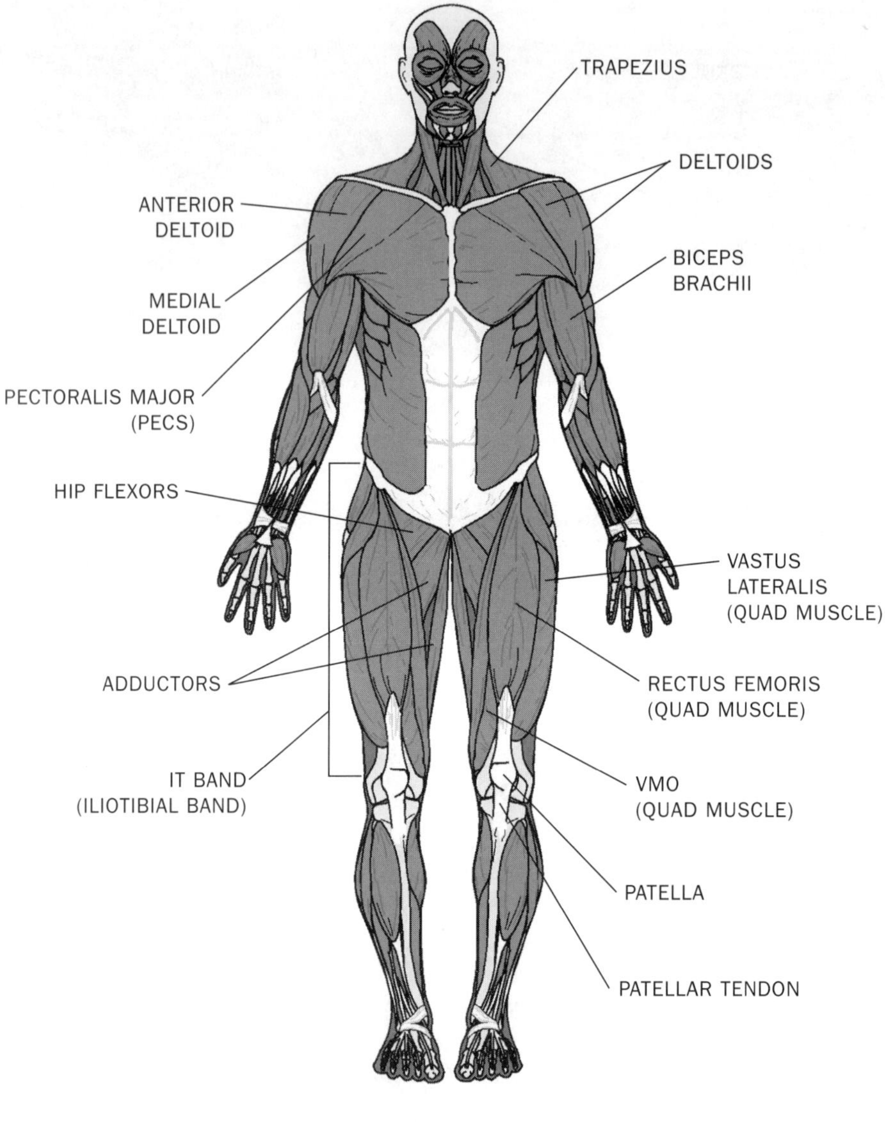
TRAPEZIUS
DELTOIDS
ANTERIOR DELTOID
BICEPS BRACHII
MEDIAL DELTOID
PECTORALIS MAJOR (PECS)
HIP FLEXORS
VASTUS LATERALIS (QUAD MUSCLE)
ADDUCTORS
RECTUS FEMORIS (QUAD MUSCLE)
IT BAND (ILIOTIBIAL BAND)
VMO (QUAD MUSCLE)
PATELLA
PATELLAR TENDON

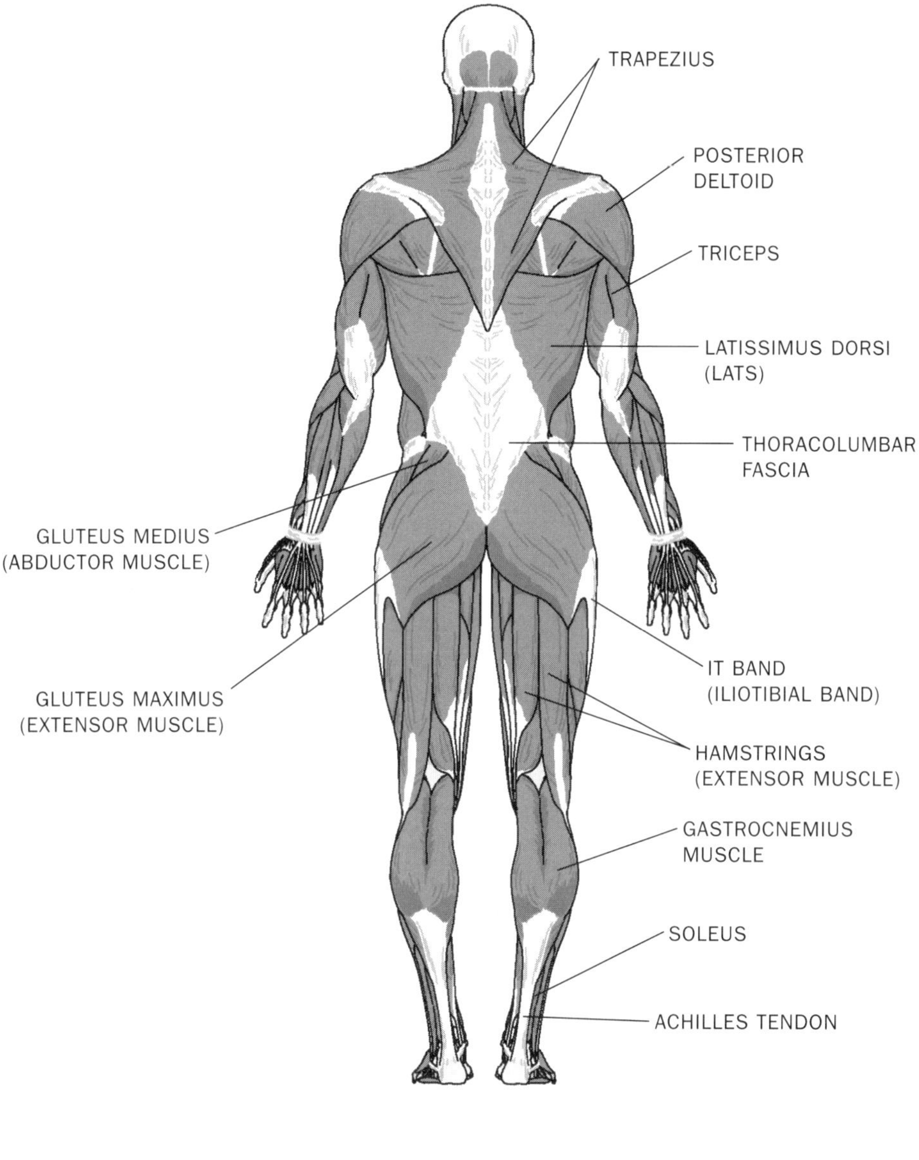
TRAPEZIUS
POSTERIOR DELTOID
TRICEPS
LATISSIMUS DORSI (LATS)
THORACOLUMBAR FASCIA
GLUTEUS MEDIUS (ABDUCTOR MUSCLE)
GLUTEUS MAXIMUS (EXTENSOR MUSCLE)
IT BAND (ILIOTIBIAL BAND)
HAMSTRINGS (EXTENSOR MUSCLE)
GASTROCNEMIUS MUSCLE
SOLEUS
ACHILLES TENDON

The Body's Response to Injury

To understand the following chapters in this book, you need to understand the basics of how the body responds to injury. With this knowledge, you will be much better equipped to tell the difference between a minor problem and an injury that is serious enough to require a trip to the emergency room.

While different injuries cause different body responses, many injuries cause inflammation of the surrounding area. Inflammation is a complicated chemical process that prepares the body for a "job." The job may be to repair a strained hamstring muscle or to form a scab over a cut on the arm. Swelling, warmth, redness, and pain characterize acute inflammation, which occurs immediately after an injury and lasts thirty-six to seventy-two hours.

Inflammation causes capillaries (tiny blood vessels) to fill with blood, producing redness and pain. Inflammation also makes the affected area warmer than other areas on the body. Blood, fluid, and other materials (such as proteins) leak from gaps in the capillaries, making the area swollen. These gaps aren't bad—they allow white blood cells to enter the injured area. This is especially important if infection causes the inflammation, because white blood cells consume bacteria and other foreign bodies. Platelets within the blood form clots, like the scabs on small skin wounds.

If the inflammation doesn't subside quickly, these cells form scar tissue. Although scar tissue is good to close a wound, too much scar tissue can cause problems. Physicians and physical therapists will often prescribe exercises that minimalize scar tissue by improving the injured region's range of motion.

Some types of injuries swell more than others. Tendons, for example, do not have a large blood supply, so tendonitis (the inflammation of tendons) typically doesn't cause a lot of swelling. A complete tendon rupture would cause more swelling than tendonitis, but not as much as a torn ligament, which has a larger blood supply.

Aiding the healing process, then, becomes your challenge. While we want the body to repair the injury, we do not want the pain and swelling that come with it. Read the Evaluation, Treatment, and Prevention chapter for specific suggestions to treat these symptoms.

The Skin: The Integumentary System

The skin is the main component of the integumentary system. In fact, the skin is the largest organ of the body and makes up 15 to 20 percent of the total body mass.

The skin has two main layers, the epidermis and the dermis. The outer layer of the epidermis is actually a layer of dead skin cells, covered with a hard protein layer. The cells are alive at the lowest level of the epidermis, which is always producing new cells underneath the old layers. As they mature, the new, living cells push the older cells to the surface of the skin. As the cells reach the outer surface, they slowly die and become hard. In fact, it takes less than one month for new skin cells to reach the outer layer, die, and slough off. Believe it or not, we lose layers of skin all the time, and our bodies keep replacing old layers with younger, newer tissue.

The epidermis forms a barrier to keep infection out, which is naturally a good feature. If this layer is intact, microorganisms cannot penetrate the skin. If the epidermis has an opening (from a scrape or a cut, for example), the exposed tissue is susceptible to infection. For that reason, letting a wound "air dry" does not hasten recovery. Bacteria and viruses attach to the skin all the time. When the skin rids itself of the outer layer, the bacteria and viruses usually go with it. This process helps prevent illness and infection. But with an opening in the epidermis, bacteria and viruses have a way in.

The epidermis also holds some sensory cells. These cells perceive touch, pressure, and pain. They pass information to the brain (through the spinal cord), and our brains respond.

The second layer of skin, the dermis, connects or anchors the epidermis to the muscles, bones, fat, and other tissue; supplies oxygen and other nutrients to the epidermis; and also contains some sensory cells.

The sweat glands and hair follicles are other important structures in the integumentary system. When the core body temperature rises, the body produces sweat, which is forced into sweat gland ducts (the tiny canals that bring sweat to the surface of the skin). As sweat evaporates, the skin temperature lowers. We have no control over the sweating mechanism, which is designed to lower our body temperature. If we try to stop the process of body cooling, we risk death. Wrestlers, for example, try to sweat excessively to lose weight. Some do this by exercising with rubber suits, which keep heat in and do not allow sweat to evaporate. Sometimes, they work past the point of heat stroke, a medical emergency that will lead to death if left untreated. (Read the Emergency Procedures chapter for more information on heat-related illnesses.)

The hair follicles, which construct hair, are alive and rich with sensory nerve endings. The hair itself is actually dead, but the growth of the hair follicles makes our hair appear to grow. That hair is dead should not be a surprise; after all, it doesn't hurt to cut our hair or nails. Living cells have nerve endings, which sense pain. The hair and nails are made up of a special kind of cell called a keratinized cell.

Just as people can get bacterial infections in their throat (strep throat), people can get skin infections. Wrestlers are at particular risk for skin infections and often acquire a fungal infection known as ringworm. It is very contagious, so proper treatment is important. If you notice a ring-like rash on your son's skin, ask your doctor to take a look at it. Other fungal infections include athlete's foot, which causes irritation and a burning sensation in the toes and might even crack the skin. Over-the-counter products like Tinactin will help the problem. Jock itch is similar to athlete's foot, but this fungal infection is near the genitals. If your son has athlete's foot, tell him to put on his socks before he puts on his underwear. Otherwise, when his underwear passes over his feet, the fabric could spread the infection from the feet to the groin. If his feet are covered, this won't happen.

Bacterial skin infections can be very contagious. An example of a bacterial infection is impetigo, which affects one person out of every thousand. Impetigo can occur on skin where there is no visible break. It begins as an itchy, red sore that first blisters, then oozes, forming a yellow crust. The fluid oozing from the blisters quickly spreads the infection. Physicians usually prescribe antibiotics to treat impetigo. Boils are another type of infection that can cause problems. If you notice a very large, very hard infection (that looks like a huge pimple), do not try to squeeze it. This may be a boil, and squeezing it may make the infection worse. Some boils require surgical excision and antibiotic medication. You can prevent most bacterial infections by washing with antibacterial soap and keeping all competitive surfaces (like wrestling mats) clean.

The skin can also play host to viral infections. Cold sores and fever blisters are examples of viral infections. They come from a strain of the herpes virus and are very contagious. People with these sores should be careful that the viral sore does not touch another person's skin. Most of these viruses are not airborne, but they spread easily, even with incidental contact. Warts are also viral infections. The papiloma virus, for example, causes plantar warts. Over-the-counter products at the local pharmacy may work with varying degrees of success. Some of these products use an acid-based medication that destroys the virus and reduces the dead skin buildup that forms the wart.

Most parents and coaches will see many skin injuries. Scraped elbows and skinned knees are almost inevitable for an active child. For instance, your daughter may suffer an abrasion on her knee or the back of her thigh if she slides into second base. Most skin injuries aren't life-threatening, but cleaning the wound is very important. The risk of infection and more serious problems increases if dirt and other foreign materials remain inside the wound. Scrub the wound gently, but thoroughly, with soap and water until it is free from dirt and other materials. Don't be concerned if the wound bleeds a little when it is scrubbed, but try to avoid using unnecessary force that might cause further injury. After cleaning, apply an antibacterial ointment and cover the wound to prevent infection.

When your hockey-playing son falls chin-first on the ice, he may have an irregular cut, or laceration, on his chin. Some lacerations require sutures (stitches), and some do not. See a physician for stitches if the wound is large or does not close easily with a normal bandage. Wounds on joints, like the elbow and the knee, often require stitches, because the skin moves and stretches every time we use the joint.

Always see a physician if an opponent's (or sibling's) teeth or mouth caused the wound. Since the human mouth is full of bacteria, your child may need antibiotic medication to prevent infection.

Any object (teeth, the tip of an ice skate, or a bike spoke, for example) can pierce the skin and cause a puncture wound. Always scrub these wounds clean to prevent infection, and see a physician if the wound was caused by a bite.

The Endocrine System

The glands in the endocrine system create and release hormones that affect other organs or tissues. Interestingly, some organs, like the liver and the pancreas, have both endocrine and exocrine functions (exocrine glands secrete a substance that is delivered to a target organ through a duct). The hormones secreted by the endocrine glands help keep the body running smoothly. A good balance of hormones is especially important for athletes. The male and female reproductive systems also contain endocrine glands. The reproductive systems are discussed in the next section.

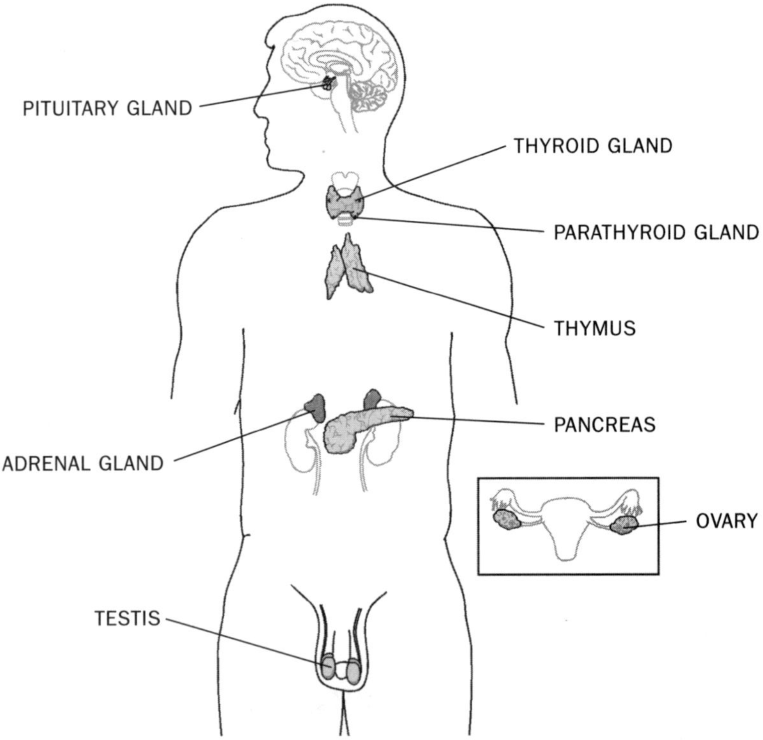

The pituitary gland, located in the brain, is the master gland of the endocrine system. This gland secretes chemicals that tell the other glands what to do. The pituitary gland controls production of the growth hormone, as well as an antidiuretic hormone that tells the kidneys to reabsorb water. Without this hormone, people would lose about twenty liters of fluid every day through urination.

The thyroid gland is positioned over the trachea, or windpipe (near the Adam's apple). It secretes hormones essential for normal growth and development. The thyroid gland is especially important for athletes because it regulates body temperature and metabolism (the rate at which our bodies use fuel). People with hypothyroidism (not enough thyroid hormone) tend to be heavyset. They also may become cold easily because they are not using sufficient fuel to maintain body heat. People with hyperthyroidism (too much thyroid hormone) are just the opposite. They tend to be thin (they usually can eat a lot of food without gaining weight) and full of energy. However, these people tend to have increased heart rates when they are at rest.

Graves' Disease is a form of hyperthyroidism in which the thyroid puts too many hormones into the system. The body responds by attacking the thyroid gland to slow the release of the thyroid hormone. When attacked, the thyroid releases more hormones, and the cycle continues. This disease can be easily treated and controlled with medication and radiation. Because the thyroid also absorbs iodine in the body, radioactive iodine often "zaps" the thyroid and stops the vicious circle. If left untreated, Graves' Disease will cause the eyes to protrude—a common sign of the disorder. Scientists do not know exactly why the eyes bulge as a result of the disease, but it is possible that the same cells that attack the thyroid also attack the tissues behind the eyes, causing inflammation and swelling. (Both former President and Mrs. Bush have Graves' Disease. If you look at a photo of Mrs. Bush, you may notice that she has swollen eyes.) People who have this disease live very normal lives. Graves' Disease is uncommon in children and adolescents.

The parathyroid glands sit behind the thyroid and produce a hormone that regulates calcium. Calcium is crucial for nervous tissue and the contraction of muscles, including our heart and diaphragm. Although the thyroid and parathyroid are endocrine glands and reside in the neck, their functions are unrelated. (Read the Issues for Girls and Women Only chapter for more information about the importance of calcium for strong bones.)

The adrenal glands sit on top of the kidneys and secrete a hormone called adrenaline. This hormone speeds metabolism and increases circulation to the muscles. Your son or daughter may experience this "adrenaline rush" during athletic activity. The adrenal glands also secrete hormones that help our kidneys regulate hydration, sodium (salt), and potassium.

The pancreas is a vital gland that secretes digestive enzymes (exocrine) and an important hormone called insulin (endocrine). Think of insulin as the key that unlocks the door to the cells in our bodies. Before the cells can use simple sugar for fuel, the sugar needs to pass from the bloodstream to the cells. The insulin "unlocks" the door, so to speak, to the cells. The cells cannot receive sugar (fuel) without this hormone. Without fuel, cells die. This is what happens to diabetes mellitus patients. If diabetic people control their sugar (food) intake and insulin levels, athletic participation is rarely a problem. Even with careful management of this disease, however, diabetic children and adults sometimes need a sugar boost. During athletic activity, muscles burn fuel so fast that sometimes the body has too much insulin, especially if the athlete has taken insulin medication. Adding sugar restores normal glucose levels. In your first-aid kit, think about packing a bag of candy or a can of orange juice. These products will have enough sugar to raise glucose levels adequately in a diabetic athlete experiencing a reaction to too much insulin.

Low glucose levels can also be a problem for non-diabetic people. Eating well throughout the day is essential for maintaining a high energy level and performing at your best. One orthopedic surgeon postponed a mid-day surgery because she was running late and didn't want to miss lunch. The doctor explained that if she didn't eat, her blood sugar would drop and she would be less than effective in the operating room. Hearing it explained this way, the patient chose to wait for an hour. The surgery went very well.

Consult your physician if you or your child has any of the following diabetes symptoms over a long period of time:

- Excessive thirst. This happens in diabetics because the body takes water away from the tissues to dissolve the sugar in the bloodstream, leading to dehydration.
- Frequent urination. This happens because simple blood sugar is filtered from the blood (by the kidneys) and enters into the urine, which causes water molecules to follow. In essence, this dehydrates the tissues.
- Unexplained irritability, weakness, and/or fatigue. This happens because of the body's lack of usable blood sugar.

Fortunately, many endocrine ailments can be managed through medication. Be certain to ask your physician if you suspect that your child has problems with normal maturation or development—he or she may have a hormone imbalance. For example, one local high-school student was obese. As you can imagine, his classmates teased him. When his physician examined his thyroid, he discovered that the young man had a metabolic disorder that could be treated with medication. The boy lost the excess weight and resumed a more normal childhood.

The Male Reproductive System

The scrotum is the loose bag of skin that holds the testicles. The testicles are endocrine glands that secrete the hormone testosterone and also produce sperm. Testosterone is the hormone that accounts for many male characteristics, such as body and facial hair, increased muscle mass, and lowered voice. Anabolic steroids are derivatives of this hormone.

The testicles house the sperm outside the body because the sperm must remain cooler than body temperature to survive. However, because the testicles are on the outside of the body, they can be easily injured (especially in contact sports). Encourage your son to wear a protective cup while playing sports like baseball and hockey.

The epididymis are the tubes that carry sperm away from the testicles. Although they appear very small, these tubes measure between four and six meters in length when uncoiled. The vas deferens are extensions of the epididymis that carry sperm to the prostate gland and seminal vesicles. This tube is cut and closed when men have vasectomies. The urethra carries the sperm out of the penis.

The prostate gland and the seminal vesicles secrete a fluid that nourishes the sperm and helps transport the sperm in ejaculation. Because the prostate surrounds the urethra (just below the bladder), urination can be painful and difficult when this gland is unhealthy or diseased. Cancer of the prostate is a concern for older men.

The penis makes fertilization possible. The penis is made up of highly erectile tissue, which enables the penis to become hard during sexual arousal. Injuries to the penis are not as common as testicular injuries. If your son has a groin injury, be concerned first about his testicles.

If your son is hit in the crotch, have him lay on his back, pull his legs to his chest, and hold them there. This eases the pain and relieves the tiny muscle spasms that occur in the genital area. Then ask him to feel his testicles. Both should feel normal. If he asks what "normal" means, tell him that they should feel like they do every morning in the shower. If one is extremely painful or extremely swollen, consult your physician immediately. Ice will reduce the pain and swelling of groin injuries. While icing the crotch sounds unpleasant, most boys and men will agree that after suffering a groin injury, the situation cannot get much worse!

One hockey goalie was struck in the groin with a puck. The puck pinched his left testicle between his protective cup and his pubic bone, damaging his testicle. Physicians ordered an ultrasound to determine if the organ would survive. Fortunately, he did not require surgery.

Because of the importance of the testicles for reproductive reasons, always consult with your physician if your son has pain or abnormal swelling. Keep in mind that the testicles can rotate within the scrotum and cut off the blood supply (known as testicular torsion). This can happen even without trauma. Testicular torsion causes excruciating pain in the groin (and occasionally in the abdominal area) and requires surgery. Left untreated, the male may lose the organ.

The Female Reproductive System

The ova (eggs) mature in the ovaries. The ovaries produce estrogen and progesterone, hormones necessary for the development of female sex organs and sex characteristics. (The importance of estrogen to the female athlete is discussed in the Issues for Girls and Women Only chapter. You may wish to review this if you have questions.) Because the ovaries are inside the body, they are protected from injury. If your daughter has severe pain that may seem like painful menstrual cramps, consult your physician. The problem may be more severe than normal menstrual cramps. Ovarian cysts, which can cause severe abdominal pain, are a possible consideration.

The fallopian tubes carry the ovum (egg) from the ovary to the uterus. The uterus is the pear-shaped muscular structure that holds a fertilized egg (embryo). If an egg is not fertilized, or an embryo is not present, the uterus sheds its lining each month. This is the female menstrual cycle. Amenorrhea, the absence of a normal menstrual cycle, is a significant problem for female athletes. (Again, see the Issues for Girls and Women Only chapter for details.)

Females have separate openings for urination and reproduction. The urethra is the small tube that carries urine from the bladder to the outside. It is located just above the vagina. The vagina is the birth canal, leading from the cervix (near the uterus) to the exterior of the body. The primary female reproductive organs are internal. However, external structures, like the labia minor and major and the clitoris, play important roles in sexuality. Injuries to these areas are rare, but possible. Consult your physician if your daughter complains of pain and notices unusual bleeding or redness in this sensitive area.

While the mammary glands do not play any role in reproduction, they are considered part of the reproductive system because they supply milk for the newborn infant. Injuries to the breasts are not usually severe, but being hit in the chest can be very painful.

The Digestive System

The food we eat goes through a complicated transformation that ultimately provides fuel for our active bodies. Without the digestive system, we have no way of giving our bodies fuel (food). To understand digestion, we follow a piece of food through the system, identifying the important anatomy along the way. In an average adult male, this system is almost twenty-nine feet long!

Inside the mouth, the cheeks and the lips keep the food in, while the teeth grind up the food. Saliva is added in the mouth. Its main function is to lubricate the food to help prevent us from choking.

The esophagus carries food from the mouth to the stomach. Normally, food has a one-way ticket to the stomach. The muscular action of swallowing typically prevents vomiting, although we have all experienced an upset stomach and the unpleasant return of what we had eaten earlier. Swallowing also keeps food from going down the trachea (windpipe).

The digestive process begins in earnest in the stomach. In this hollow organ, food is mixed with digestive enzymes and hydrochloric acid. (People with bulimia lose the enamel on their teeth because the stomach acid destroys the enamel when they induce vomiting.) When the stomach is full, it is distended. Playing with a full stomach is not advantageous. During exercise, the body directs its energy to working muscles as well as the heart and lungs. The digestive process slows down during exercise.

The time food spends in the stomach varies according to the type of food. Red meat, for example, takes longer to digest than fruit. Once it is broken down, the food travels to the small intestine. The food is absorbed (creating fuel and energy for active people) in the small intestine. For the average adult male, this tube, if uncoiled, would be about nineteen feet long.

The large intestine, also called the colon, is much bigger in diameter than the small intestine, although it is not as long. The purpose of the large intestine is to absorb water from the material that is passed from the small intestine. If illness prevents the colon from absorbing water, diarrhea is the unpleasant result. The rectum is the narrowing end of the colon, and the anus is the final hole through which feces passes. The rectum is controlled by muscular tissue that allows people to control (for the most part) when they eliminate waste. Involuntary smooth-muscle contractions move the foodstuff through the system.

While most athletes won't injure their intestines, illness can disrupt the normal digestive process and may complicate athletic activity. (You can imagine how difficult it would be to compete in a sport if you needed to take a bathroom break every few minutes.) If your child has persistent diarrhea, passes blood in his or her stool, or complains of severe abdominal cramping or pain, contact your physician.

Cardiovascular System

Our muscles and tissues need oxygen to survive. The cardiovascular system (the arteries, veins, heart, lungs, and their components) transfers oxygen from the air we breathe to the blood. Through exercise, we can train our cardiovascular system to deliver oxygen-rich blood more effectively to working muscles and tissues. With training, the heart can pump more blood through the system, bringing more oxygen to the muscles, which are then able to do more work. Cardiovascular training also helps the lungs exchange carbon dioxide and oxygen more efficiently.

After the blood passes through the lungs and picks up oxygen for the rest of the body, it travels through the arteries away from the heart. Small arteries are called arterioles and small arterioles are called capillaries. Injuries to major arteries are life-threatening. As discussed in the Emergency Procedures chapter, if a wound spurts blood, call 911. This could indicate an arterial bleed that needs immediate medical attention.

Veins carry the blood that has passed through the tissues, delivering its oxygen supply and picking up carbon dioxide (the waste product of our tissues). Veins bring the blood back to the heart, where it is pumped through the lungs to pick up more oxygen from the air we breathe. The smaller veins are called venioles.

Red blood cells are the cells in the blood that carry oxygen. Proteins in red blood cells combine with iron in the body to form hemoglobin. It is this hemoglobin that actually carries the oxygen. A low iron level means that the body doesn't have enough hemoglobin to transport oxygen during exercise. If your child has a low hemoglobin level, he or she may be unable to finish practices or games without becoming completely exhausted. Sometimes, coaches mistake this condition for laziness. Always instruct your child to tell you if he or she feels abnormally winded after practice or if simple activities, such as shopping or walking up stairs, make him or her tired. This is especially true for menstruating adolescents, who lose a fair amount of blood each month through their menstrual periods. Hemoglobin fluctuations are uncommon in healthy children. Loss of blood through surgical procedures or because of internal bleeding—like a stomach ulcer—is a common cause. If you suspect that your son or daughter has low hemoglobin, consult your doctor. The solution may be as simple as increasing his or her iron intake (iron is found abundantly in red meat as well as beans and other legumes). Iron is an important element in the hemoglobin molecule.

White blood cells fight disease by consuming foreign materials, like bacteria. They also clean up damaged tissue, like when we strain our muscles, so the body can lay down new, undamaged tissue.

When your son cuts his finger, platelets form a natural bandage, clotting the blood. Platelet counts can decrease in females just before menstruation. Other causes for low platelet counts include high doses of penicillin, consumption of aspirin and other anti-inflammatories, and a genetic disease called Von Willerbrand's Disease.

People with low platelet counts should avoid contact sports. Erin suffered a nosebleed when she collided with another player during a soccer game. Because her nose would not stop bleeding, she went to the doctor. Once her nosebleed was stopped, the doctor tested her platelet count. Not surprisingly, it was tremendously low. Erin missed a few weeks of the season while her platelet count returned to normal.

The heart is divided into four chambers: two atria and two ventricles. The ventricles are bigger and pump blood out of the heart. The atria pump blood into the ventricles.

Blood enters the heart in the right atrium. The right atrium pumps blood to the right ventricle. The ventricle pumps the blood through the pulmonary artery to the lungs. The blood picks up oxygen and travels back to the heart through the pulmonary vein. The left atrium receives the blood and then pumps it to the left ventricle. The left ventricle (which is by far the largest of the four chambers) pumps the blood through the aorta to the rest of the body. When the heart works properly, the atria pump together and the ventricles pump together.

Between each chamber, one-way valves prevent the blood from going back into the chamber from where it was just pumped. If these valves ever fail, small amounts of blood can leak back into the previous chamber. This problem can cause dizziness or faintness. Always let a medical professional know about these symptoms.

The left lung has two lobes, and the right lung has three (the heart occupies the space on the left side where the third lobe sits on the right side). Tiny sacs in the lungs called alveoli fill with oxygen as we breathe. As blood passes through these sacs, oxygen is exchanged with carbon dioxide. The carbon dioxide, along with the inhaled oxygen that the blood did not absorb, is released when we exhale.

Air travels in and out of the lungs through the trachea and the bronchial tubes. These tubes spread out from the main air passage like branches on a tree. When people are choking, physicians sometimes do a tracheotomy, creating a hole in the trachea.

Bronchial tubes may also suffer problems. One wrestler suffered a bronchial spasm during a match and had tremendous difficulty breathing. We called an ambulance because we feared he would need an artificial airway to help him breathe. Bronchial spasms can be caused by allergic reactions, such as an allergic reaction to bee stings. Other possible causes include traumatic injuries and asthma attacks. These bronchial problems often require immediate attention.

Asthma is a lung condition that affects many children and adults. While an asthma attack can be caused by a variety of triggers, we know that some people suffer from exercise-induced asthma, a condition that makes breathing very difficult and causes tightness in the chest during and after exercise. Asthma is very treatable with medication. Call your physician if you suspect your child or player may have some form of asthma.

The Skeletal System

Our muscles and bones work together to help us run, walk, kick a ball, and do other activities. We can injure these tissues when we are active. As you read about specific muscles and bones throughout this book, refer to the illustrations on pages 4 through 7. The following general overview will help you understand the basic parts of the skeletal system.

Bones can be grouped into several types. Long bones include the femur, or the thighbone. Short bones are bones of similar size in height, width, and depth, like the carpal bones in the wrist. Flat bones are actually thin bones, like the bones that form the skull. Irregular bones include some of the facial bones. Sesamoid bones are bones within tendons, like the patellar tendon in the kneecap. Injuries to bones hurt. Broken bones cause a lot of bleeding and bruising because bones have a rich blood supply. Many athletes and parents ask the difference between a "fracture" and a "break." There is NO difference. If your son fractures his finger, he has broken his finger. If he has broken his finger, he has fractured his finger.

The ends of long bones grow together at a site called the epiphysis. This is the "growth plate" you may have heard about. Injuries to the growth plate can be serious, so you will want to seek medical advice if you suspect your son or daughter may have a growth plate fracture. You need to worry about growth plate fractures when an injury causes pain at the end of a long bone—like in the wrist, lower leg, arm, or elbow. Not every fracture injures the growth plate.

Tendons attach muscles to bones. We can strain (and sometimes tear) muscles and tendons. Because tendons do not have the same type of blood supply as muscles, the body does not have a quick and easy way to heal its tendons. Therefore, tendonitis (inflammation of the tendon) injuries can take some time to heal. Although athletes with tendonitis experience pain with activity, there is usually not a lot of swelling. Remember, inflammation and swelling are not the same thing. Inflammation is one way the body responds to injury—it adds heat to increase blood circulation to the injury. Swelling, on the other hand, is a collection of fluid that occurs as a direct result of an injury.

Ice, anti-inflammatory medication, and strengthening exercises are good treatments for tendon injuries. Young athletes with tendonitis will probably not suffer permanent damage if they continue to play. However, if the pain becomes so severe that it interferes with daily activities (like walking up and down the stairs or brushing their teeth in the morning), it is time to see a doctor.

Ligaments help stabilize joints by connecting bones to other bones. We sprain ligaments. Parents and athletes often ask, "Did I sprain it or just tear it a little?" Both! A sprain is a tear. The degree of the sprain refers to the severity of the tear. In other words, a minor sprain involves a minor tear of the ligament tissue. Unlike tendon injuries, ligament sprains may cause a lot of swelling. For example, when the anterior cruciate ligament in the knee is injured, there is usually a lot of swelling within an hour after the incident. (For more on this ligament, see the Knee chapter.)

Ligament sprains can vary in intensity. Some sprains can be minor and some can be very serious. Your physician may refer to these as Grade-I, Grade-II, or Grade-III injuries. Grade-I injuries are very minor; Grade-III injuries indicate that the ligament is completely torn or severed. Ligament injuries often make the joint feel unstable. When a ligament is injured, strengthening the muscles around the joint can make up for lost stability. Ice, strengthening the injured area, and improving range of motion are good treatments for patients with these injuries. Focus initial treatment on controlling pain and swelling (see page 124) and improving range of motion. If you think your child might have a ligament injury, talk to a physical therapist or an athletic trainer for advice on specific exercises.

Kids young and old will experience strained muscles. You may hear someone say that he or she has "pulled" a hamstring. A pulled hamstring is the same as a strained hamstring. Fortunately, muscles are rich with blood vessels, so they heal quickly. However, they also tend to bleed when they are damaged. Serious muscle strains cause bruising and discoloration. Use ice, stretching, and strengthening exercises to treat these strains. A physical therapist or certified athletic trainer will be able to give you specific ideas for your child's case.

A bursa sac (the plural is "bursae") is a small, fluid-filled sac that protects tendons and muscles, reducing friction over bones. Inflamed bursae cause pain, and some can become extremely swollen. In the case of the olecranon bursa sac (see page 184), acute inflammation makes the elbow look like Popeye's elbow. Ice, compression, and anti-inflammatory medication usually work well to treat this type of injury.

The Nervous System

The nervous system is very complex and is made up of many different components. The brain and the spinal cord make up the central nervous system (CNS), which is the command center of the body. Information travels from the brain down the spinal cord and on to other parts of the body. The peripheral nervous system is composed of the nerves that connect to the CNS and other individual nerves. Parts of the peripheral nervous system include the twelve cranial nerves (nerves inside the head) and the spinal nerves (which branch off the spinal cord).

The peripheral nervous system has afferent and efferent divisions. The afferent nerves, or sensory nerves, carry information from receptors in the skin and from the organs in the body. The efferent nerves carry information to muscles. We can choose to send some of these messages (like when our brain tells our muscles to contract as we lift something), while some messages are sent automatically (like when our heart beats or our intestines push food through the digestive process).

Injuries to nerves can be drastic. If your child ever has unexplained weakness or tingling in the arms, hands, legs, or feet, contact your physician immediately. A physician can perform tests to determine if a person has nerve damage. One such test is called an EMG (which stands for electromyelogram). This test can determine which nerve is damaged and to what extent. Nerve injuries can be caused by contusion injuries, overstretching, or pressure from herniated disks in the neck or lower back. Some common symptoms of nerve injuries include weakness, numbness, radiating pain, and burning or tingling in the extremities.

Musculoskeletal Differences between Males and Females

Although there are not many physical differences between the sexes, subtle differences in anatomical structure may be related to certain injuries in some female athletes. Physicians, physical therapists, and athletic trainers throughout the country are engaging in constructive discussions regarding these topics, but conclusions still vary from one professional to the next.

One of the most commonly discussed injury areas for girls and women is the knee. Females have a higher Q-angle than males do. The easiest way to imagine the Q-angle is to picture the angle formed by the intersection of the femur (thigh) and the tibia (shin).

Women have higher Q-angles for several reasons:

- The female hips are wider. All adolescent females go through a natural process in which their hips widen as their bodies prepare for possible childbirth. When adolescent female athletes experience knee pain, clinical evaluation often shows an increased Q-angle.
- Females tend to have more medial stress than males do. In nonprofessional terms, this is sometimes referred to as being "knock-kneed."

To what, then, does this predispose your young daughter? Well, that depends largely on the sports your daughter participates in. For athletes involved in jumping or pivoting sports, like basketball or soccer, most people agree that the rate of ACL tears (discussed in the Knee chapter) is higher among females. Although a relationship may exist between Q-angle and certain knee injuries, research has not proven this. Young women who participate in other sports do not seem as at risk as soccer- and basketball-playing girls.

Another possible correlation with ACL tears involves the ovulation cycle. ACL tears seem to occur more often in athletes who are ovulating. Ovulation causes hormonal changes, and some professionals feel that women are at greater risk for injury during ovulation. Again, this has not been proven, but some researchers feel the subject is an important issue worthy of further research. (These same researchers do *not* recommend that you withhold your daughter from competition while she ovulates.)

Another knee injury that young women typically encounter is patellofemoral joint syndrome (kneecap injury), which is also discussed in the Knee chapter. Again, whether or not Q-angle is the culprit for this injury is under discussion in the medical community. While people in the sports medicine field seem to see more patellar dislocations in the female population, research does not support this claim. However, as the Q-angle increases, more lateral stress is placed on the kneecap (patella), which could cause a dislocation.

Certainly, the Q-angle could cause the kneecap to be aligned incorrectly, which can contribute to patellofemoral joint pain and other overuse injuries. Your physician will be able to determine if your daughter's knee pain is related to the alignment of her kneecap.

How, then, do we prevent these injuries? Some injuries are difficult to prevent because they involve acute, traumatic events.

However, there are preventative steps your daughter can take to avoid knee injuries:

- Encourage her to strengthen her quadriceps (the muscles in the front of her thigh) and her hamstrings (the muscles in the back). Some people feel that there is a tendency for young women to strengthen only their quadriceps muscles and neglect their hamstrings. It is important to strike a balance between these two muscle groups. Contact an athletic trainer in your area for specific suggestions regarding this.
- Wear appropriate footwear for competitions. This is good prevention for both men and women. Some people feel that there are structural differences between men's and women's feet, and that appropriate gear is necessary.
- Encourage conditioning. It is no secret that as fatigue sets in, people are at higher risk for injury. Encourage your young daughter to maintain adequate conditioning levels throughout the season.

The Elbow and Shoulder

Girls and young women have a higher carrying angle than boys and young men do. The carrying angle is the angle formed by the humerus and radius/ulna when an individual's arm hangs at his or her side, palm facing forward. Because the carrying angle for women is between five and ten degrees higher than that of men, some professionals feel that young women are at risk for injuries to the elbow. This is especially true if they participate in softball or racquet sports.

Research has not proven this, however, and we do not want to imply that your daughter will have an injury, such as medial epicondylitis (discussed in the Elbow, Wrist, and Hand chapter), because her elbow has a larger carrying angle than her brother's. We are simply suggesting that if your daughter develops one of these injuries, she may have been predisposed because of her structure. Contact your physician if you have any questions regarding this.

Some medical professionals feel that females, especially swimmers, are predisposed to shoulder injury because of two factors:

- Females sometimes have shorter limbs than males. This means that they may have to take more strokes to swim the same distance as their male counterparts. As their strokes increase, so does their risk of shoulder injuries like impingement syndrome, rotator cuff tendonitis, and bursitis. (See the Shoulder chapter.)
- Females in our society are often discouraged from strengthening their upper bodies. Admittedly, this is more of a social issue than a structural one, but, certainly, strength is one way to prevent these injuries.

To prevent injuries, your most important job as a parent or coach is to teach proper techniques for running, swimming, kicking, throwing, lifting, and any other activities your child's sport requires. In addition, encourage girls and young women to strengthen their bodies. Strong bodies promote not only athletic success, but also healthy lifestyles and high self-esteem. Contact an athletic trainer or physical therapist for specific strengthening exercises for your young daughter.

The Foot and Ankle

Some young women have a wide forefoot and a narrow hindfoot. This may create a problem for your daughter as she tries to find shoes. Poorly fitted shoes cause injuries.

While some women may be more prone to foot and ankle injuries than men, the reasons are often more social that structural. As your daughter matures and goes to formal dances like the prom, she will likely wear high-heeled shoes.

High-heeled shoes can be a source of injury for several reasons:

- High-heeled shoes place the ankle in a position that is vulnerable to ankle sprains.
- High-heeled shoes lift the heel, causing tightness in the Achilles tendon. If your daughter wears high-heeled shoes a lot, she should stretch her Achilles tendon before she participates in athletics.
- Formal dress shoes tend to predispose the foot to bunions and other injuries (discussed in the Foot, Ankle, Lower Leg, and Toe chapter).

Conclusion

We do not have space here to discuss every part of the body. For example, we have not discussed the kidneys or the urinary system. Some information on these topics can be found in the Issues for Girls and Women Only chapter. We have not discussed the spleen, an organ that manufactures red blood cells. Injuries to this organ are covered in the Emergency Procedures chapter. Spleen injuries are serious. The spleen removes iron from the hemoglobin of red blood cells. A malfunctioning spleen may increase its normal rate of destroying red blood cells, resulting in different types of anemia. The spleen is so rich with blood that an injury can also cause excessive blood loss. Refer to the Emergency Procedures chapter for what to do in case of an internal organ injury. The Emergency Procedures chapter also discusses injuries to the liver. The liver's role in energy storage is reviewed in the Exercise, Conditioning, and Nutrition chapter.

Frequently Asked Questions

Q: *My fourteen-year-old daughter and I are having a debate over sunscreen. She thinks only older sunbathers get skin cancer. I say that if she is playing tennis outside in the sun every day, she is at risk. Who is right? Does she need sunscreen or not?*

A: You are right. She needs sunscreen, badly. In fact, one young high-school tennis player recently had a cancerous tumor removed from her forehead. She played tennis every day in the summer and never wore sunscreen. She was, I am sure, much like your daughter. She thought she was invincible. Fortunately, doctors discovered and removed her tumor in time. She will likely never have another scare.

Q: *My eleven-year-old son and I are having a discussion over how much fluid he should drink a day. I say that he should drink several glasses of water per day. He wants to drink nothing but Gatorade. How can I be certain that he is getting enough fluid?*

A: Tell him that he may drink his Gatorade (provided you are willing to buy it for him) on one condition: he must check the color of his urine when he goes to the bathroom. If it is not clear, he needs to drink more water or Gatorade. This is a good test for all athletes. Dark urine (dark yellow or gold) indicates dehydration; clear urine indicates adequate fluid levels. Although this is not an issue families bring up around the dinner table, it is a great way of knowing how much water a person should drink.

Q: *My daughter has a hard time breathing, but only when she plays soccer. Does she have allergies? Why would she have such a hard time?*

A: We will make two assumptions here. First, we assume your daughter has this problem only when she exercises. Second, we will assume that your daughter is in otherwise good health, with no heart problems. She may have exercise-induced asthma. This form of asthma only appears during exercise, but is treated in the same way as other types of asthma. Contact your doctor, explain the situation, and ask if an inhaler would be appropriate for your daughter.

Q: *My son wakes up every night in a cold sweat and has been feeling dizzy lately. He is also going to the bathroom a lot. What do you think this means?*

A: Your son may have diabetes. Talk to your doctor about what you have noticed. If your son has diabetes, stay positive. Many athletes do just fine if they control their medication and watch what they eat and drink. Keep in mind that nighttime sweats may also indicate something mores serious than diabetes. Contact your doctor.

Q: *My dad used to say that a fracture is worse than a sprain. Is he right?*

A: Yes and no. This depends on the type of fracture and the type of sprain. It also depends on which bone is broken and which ligament is sprained. For example, some fractures are so serious that surgeons must use screws and metal plates to hold the bone together. Some sprains are so serious that physicians must surgically repair them. In general, ligaments provide stability to joints. Tearing (which is the same as spraining) a ligament can cause long-term instability in the joint if left untreated. While sprained ligaments require daily exercises, icing, and other long-term therapies, most simple fractures require only time to heal.

Contributing Author: Jim Hackney, MHS, PT

Jim is a physical therapist with the Institute for Athletic Medicine, Osseo Clinic, where he also serves as Clinic Supervisor. Jim treats a variety of sports and orthopedic patients. He lettered in wrestling for four years at Marquette University. Jim is currently enrolled in a doctoral studies program in Kinesiology at the University of Minnesota. He and his wife, Mary, live in Maple Grove, Minnesota.

Chapter

2

Exercise, Conditioning, and Nutrition for the Young Athlete

Every expert seems to recommend a different method for exercising and getting in shape, and most libraries and bookstores have shelves of material supporting a variety of exercise and conditioning theories. All this information can be confusing for the average person.

In this chapter, we hope to dispel some common myths about exercise, conditioning, and nutrition. If you have further questions about anything you read here, contact your physician or an athletic trainer. As always, your child should consult a physician before beginning any conditioning program (many schools require annual physical exams for children who participate in athletic activities). Your doctor can offer advice and make suggestions about a program that is safe for your athlete.

What Is Physical Fitness?

Physical fitness involves more than being strong or running three miles every day. In fact, true physical fitness includes four components—strength, flexibility, agility, and endurance. To be truly physically fit, athletes must work to improve their ability in all these areas. Most people only dedicate time to one or two of these areas in their quest for fitness. A combination of all these components, however, will reduce the risk of injury and improve athletic performance.

Strength

Strength is the ability to exert a force (when doing a pull-up or push-up, for example) or withstand a stress (like a guard in football blocking his opponent). When speaking of strength, bigger does not mean better. Many young high-school males seem to think that chest and arm strength are the keys to physical fitness, and they will often ignore the other components of fitness.

Gaining strength does not always require weight lifting or daily trips to the gym. Tom, a high-school hockey player, wanted to improve his strength, so he decided to do ten push-ups and ten sit-ups every hour of the day. This took only a few minutes out of each hour, and he thought he could do it easily. At the end of the first day, Tom was sore. His muscles were working harder than usual. By the end of the week, he was doing 140 to 160 push-ups and sit-ups per day. He felt stronger. He lost the flab, as he called it, around his abdomen and arms. He felt better about himself, and he didn't spend a lot of money on a club membership.

Flexibility

Flexibility is perhaps the most overlooked component of fitness. It can have a profound impact on injury prevention. Flexibility can also improve your performance, keeping muscles stretched and limber. Muscle tissue is elastic by nature, and muscles tend to shorten as they get stronger (which is why professional football linemen are inherently less flexible than running backs, for example). Ask a physician or athletic trainer to show you a few stretching exercises for you and your child.

The key to flexibility training is to maintain a consistent routine. Stretching every day is easy to do and requires very little time or special equipment. You do not need an expensive health club membership to stretch major muscle groups. When high-school athletes tell us they didn't have time to stretch, we always ask about the television programs they watched the night before. If they have time to watch TV, they have time to stretch. Commercials are a great time for stretching and simple strengthening exercises. Becoming fit doesn't have to be time consuming or difficult. After all, even five minutes of gentle stretching is better than no stretching at all.

Agility

Agility is the ability to perceive your body in relation to the playing surface. Making quick stops and starts and maintaining balance are skills that demand agility. Gymnasts, ice skaters, and even football players use agility in their sports. The skills developed by agility training will greatly improve athletic performance. Again, talk to a doctor or athletic trainer about basic agility drills.

Endurance

Endurance is the ability to perform a physical activity for an extended period of time at a steady or constant level. Marathon runners, for example, have great endurance. Like Forrest Gump, they can run for a very long time. Elite marathon runners require slightly over two hours to run twenty-six miles. Soccer players may run three to five miles in a single game without a rest. Hockey players, on the other hand, usually only skate in shifts of thirty to forty-five seconds. These athletes may not have the endurance of a cross-country runner or a soccer player.

Building endurance strengthens the muscles, the heart, and the lungs. Muscles gain endurance if they need to work over an extended period of time. Endurance helps the heart and lungs supply the muscles with the fuel and oxygen they need to perform for extended periods.

Frequently Asked Questions

Q: *What can my young daughter do to get in shape? Does she need to do something specific in each of the four categories?*

A: General play is great for most young children. Encourage children to play tag and hide-and-seek with other children. If no other children are present, general play is good for adults, too! Preteens are too young for a formal conditioning program, and general play promotes physical growth, social interaction with other children, and the development of good habits for later in life.

Encourage your child to be active in extra-curricular activities. Even non-sport-related activities promote social interaction and require some effort from your child. Think of it as addition by subtraction: If your daughter is doing something productive, she is not in front of the television!

Q: *What makes football and cross-country running so different? Why do children need to prepare differently for them?*

A: Earlier, we mentioned that endurance was a component of fitness. Distance running and swimming require a lot of endurance, but football does not. Each play in football lasts only a few seconds. Even if someone runs one hundred yards for a touchdown, the play only lasts fifteen to twenty seconds.

This highlights the difference between anaerobic and aerobic sports. Anaerobic sports (meaning "without oxygen") require short bursts of energy, like in football, wrestling, and weight lifting. Athletes who participate in anaerobic sports us less oxygen in their athletic activities than those involved in aerobic sports, but they are visibly winded afterward. You probably don't breathe heavily as you sprint a short distance, for example.

Aerobic sports (meaning "with oxygen"), on the other hand, require a great deal of breathing during the activity. You would breathe quite a lot during a two-mile run. Examples of aerobic sports are distance running, distance swimming, and bicycling.

Therefore, if a child wants to run cross-country or swim distance events, he or she will need to focus on endurance activities, such as running, swimming, or biking. If he or she wants to play rugby or ice hockey, which are anaerobic activities, your child should first focus on strength and agility exercises, then endurance.

Q: *When is it safe for my child to begin working with a personal fitness trainer?*

A: Generally, children can begin formal workouts when they reach age fifteen or sixteen. Even then, they are not completely ready for all types of work. Heavy weight training can greatly affect bone growth and disrupt the normal maturation process in adolescents. Consult your physician for advice on specific activities for your son or daughter.

Q: *My son wants to lift weights with his friends. What are some do's and don'ts?*

A: Assuming he is physically ready for this activity, keep the following in mind.

Low-weight, high-repetition lifting will improve strength without increasing bulk. This is ideal for adolescents because it promotes strength and does not overly stress joints and other tissues. Depending on the specific lift, twenty pounds lifted thirty times will be better than sixty pounds lifted ten times.

Always lift with a friend, especially at first. If your son should injure himself during a lift, a friend can provide help if needed. In addition, it promotes social interaction and encourages the children to remain active.

Start slow. Jumping into an activity too fast can cause injury. Troy Aikman does not throw a thousand passes on his first day of training camp, and your child should not attempt to bench-press one hundred pounds on his first or second day of weight training. This will probably lead to an injury.

Keep in mind the do's and don'ts of weight lifting:

Do...

- Consult an expert who can teach the proper technique for all lifts. Proper technique is the key!
- Inhale while lifting. Exhale on release.
- Use a moderate and controlled speed.
- Perform the lifts through the entire range of motion.
- Keep abdominal muscles tight to support the back and trunk.

Do not...

- Rock or arch the back to lift more weight or do more repetitions.
- Try to set speed records in the weight room. Lifting correctly will increase the benefits.
- Guess what lifts you should do. Not knowing what to do can be harmful.

Q: *My son has been reading about supplements. Are they safe?*

A: It depends on the supplement. Anabolic steroids, which are synthetic forms of testosterone, are terribly unsafe. Amino acid supplements (amino acids are the building blocks of muscles) are not as harmful as steroids, but they are wasteful for an adolescent athlete. A well-balanced diet that includes adequate sources of protein and carbohydrates will provide everything an aspiring young athlete needs to be big and strong.

Q: *What should we look for if we think our son has used or is using steroids?*

A: To gain the desired effects from anabolic steroids, athletes must use them in conjunction with a strenuous weight-lifting program. Athletes who are using "correctly" will get big quickly. If you have noticed your son adding bulk to his frame in a short period time, be suspicious.

Look for the following signs if you think your son or daughter is using steroids:

- Users have wild mood swings. Minor inconveniences can make them very irritable, even hostile. One athlete ripped a paper towel dispenser off the wall and threw it into the toilet because the telephone was busy at his parent's house and he needed a ride home. This is called a "roid rage."
- Male users often have premature male-pattern baldness. High-school students typically do not lose their hair without a significant genetic reason. If your son's hair is thinning rapidly, be suspicious.

- Users get acne on their back. This is more than just an occasional pimple; it is severe and will often leave scars.
- Users often have higher rates of tendonitis and other inflammatory injuries. Very powerful muscles will stress the tendons that attach them to the bones. (It is like using a piece of twine to tow a big boat.) Be concerned if your son constantly complains of tendonitis in his shoulders or knees.
- Users often suffer from other disorders. Your son would certainly not appreciate a question about his testicles, but one sign of steroid use is a decrease in testicle size. (Female users experience a growth of the clitoris.)

If you suspect your child is using steroids, consult your physician immediately. Doctors have linked liver disease and cancer to steroid use. Continued use can cause irreversible damage, even death.

Q: *My daughter wants to buy those fluid-replacement drinks for basketball practice. Are they worthwhile?*

A: For many high-caliber, elite athletes, these drinks are both necessary and beneficial for two reasons. First, they replace the fluids lost while sweating. Fluid levels are critical to both health and performance. We would never drive a car without oil in the engine or coolant in the radiator, and we should never compete without replacing the fluids we lose through sweat. Second, fluid-replacement drinks provide calories. Our bodies use calories as energy during competitions, much like a car uses gasoline.

A logical question would be, "Does my child need a product like Gatorade?" Truthfully, the answer is no. Water is an excellent way to replenish fluids, and orange or apple slices provide the same calories as these drinks do. Some people, however, find that athletes drink these products more faithfully than water, perhaps because many young children consider it a novelty.

Q: *What foods would be good for my children to eat before their meets?*

A: Typically, we recommend foods that are high in energy and low in fat. Fatty foods are difficult for the body to digest, while carbohydrates like bread, grain, and pasta provide quick energy and are easily digested. Fruits and vegetables are also good sources of energy before a competition.

Carbohydrates can be stored in the liver and used later as the body needs them. Children require a lot of energy to grow, learn, and remain active. It is important that they have enough calories to do so.

Q: *Is it possible for my child to overtrain or exercise too much?*

A: Yes. During normal workouts, the body breaks down tissue and builds new, stronger tissue. This is how we get stronger and how our bodies adapt to the work that we demand of it. However, the body needs time to repair damaged tissue. Overuse injuries, such as tendonitis, stress fractures, and shin splints, happen when the body cannot recover quickly enough. People often reinjure themselves because they do not give their bodies a chance to recuperate. Balancing recovery time and practice time can be difficult. If you suspect that your child may be overtraining, look for changes in performance and attitude.

For young children, decreased performance may not be apparent. However, if Johnny normally scores three goals in a hockey game, and now he cannot stand on his skates, think about giving him some rest. Changes in attitude may be more noticeable than changes in performance. When volleyball was fun for your daughter, she excelled. If she has overtrained, she may not find enjoyment in the sport. If you suspect your child may be overtraining, consider giving him or her a break from athletics or activity. Remember that more is not always better.

Q: *What kinds of nutritional concerns should I have for my always-active teenage daughter?*

A: Your daughter has the same basic requirements as any other athlete. Well-balanced meals, foods that are high in carbohydrates and low in fat, plenty of fluids, and adequate intake of proteins are the fundamentals.

Female athletes are at risk for iron deficiency, which can trigger anemia. Anemia can have the same result as low hemoglobin levels (see page 19). Encourage your active daughter to consume iron-rich foods like red meat, beans and other legumes, bread, pasta, cereal, prunes, and raisins.

Protein is also very important. Girls and women often don't get enough of it. Protein is in red meat, beans and other legumes, and eggs.

Another key component in a female's diet is calcium, which is important for strong bones. Calcium is found in milk; cheese; yogurt; fish; green, leafy vegetables; and fruits like oranges and papaya. Vitamin D helps the body store calcium.

Finally, make sure that your daughter is eating enough. Many athletic young women don't eat enough. Encourage your daughter to "eat to compete."

Conclusion

Improving one's conditioning can involve high-tech and scientific principles. It can also involve minor lifestyle changes that bring remarkable results. For example, encouraging your child to play outside with friends is a great way to help him or her "stay in shape." You'd be amazed at how much healthier your child will be through simple play.

However, sports sometimes require different types of conditioning. Always keep this in mind when you encourage more formalized training. Would it be a good idea for a football team to run five miles every day? Certainly not. Would it be a good idea for a distance runner to run sprints every day? Certainly not. Design a young athlete's training and conditioning around the sports and activities the child most enjoys.

As parents and coaches, always consider the following with respect to conditioning programs:

- Time of year. Your out-of-season program should include more strength training than your in-season program. Athletes will gain strength during the off-season and maintain it throughout the season.
- The goals. What do you want your child or player to accomplish? Do you want your running back to be fast,

or do you want him to be able to run ten miles in record speed? You would probably stress speed and quickness (agility) over endurance.

- More is not always better. The body requires time to rebuild. For this reason, your daughter will have better results strengthening her quads if she does "quad exercises" every other day rather than every day. It is possible to overtrain.
- The age of your athlete or child. Younger children (under fourteen years old) have less mature bones and muscles. Students in eighth grade are more ready to begin a light strengthening program than younger kids are. Never push kids too fast—serious injury can result.

Encourage children to develop good habits early on. The best way to do this is to "practice what you preach." Parents and coaches can do a lot to promote healthy lifestyles by encouraging athletic activity, providing well-balanced meals, and approaching fitness with common sense.

Contributing Author: Jim Rakow, ATC/R

Jim is a certified athletic trainer with the Institute for Athletic Medicine, Eden Prairie Clinic. Jim is consistently one of the busiest athletic trainers throughout the IAM clinic system. He is also the Head Athletic Trainer for Bloomington Kennedy High School, a position he has held for three years. Jim is very active in the Minnesota Athletic Trainers' Association's Public Relations Committee and was instrumental in the formation of IAM's HealthClub Referral Program. Jim and his wife, Holly, live in Bloomington, Minnesota.

With Appreciation: Susie Oster, PT

Chapter 3

Evaluation, Treatment, and Prevention of Athletic Injuries

Your son comes home from football practice one evening. First, you notice that his left shoe is untied, and then you see that his ankle is swollen. What do you do?

Or imagine that you are coaching your daughter's soccer team. One of your players twists her knee. At first, you don't think it will be serious—after all, she's just a kid. Then you notice she is unable to walk without limping. What do you do?

When you are the first person to know about an injury, treating the injured child becomes your responsibility. This can be stressful, complicated, and even frightening for many parents and coaches. However, all parents and coaches can learn the basic skills necessary to recognize and evaluate injuries and provide proper, immediate care.

At many high schools, certified athletic trainers work with athletes to prevent, care for, and rehabilitate injuries. Having a certified athletic trainer on staff can reassure parents and provide a tremendous service to the schools and/or sports teams. However, this does not shield athletes from injury. Without the support of an athletic trainer, some high schools—and many junior-high and middle-school athletic programs—rely on coaches to provide medical care. Youth sports programs depend on parents and coaches for medical care. In many cases, parents and coaches are not properly trained to handle a child's injuries. This chapter explains the basic techniques for evaluating, treating, and preventing athletic injuries.

Immediate Evaluation

The body responds in many different ways when an injury occurs. Its first instinct is to protect itself. Muscles spasm and tighten to create a natural splint, preventing further injury to ligaments, tendons, and bones. This natural splint will often mask an injury, making it difficult to identify.

Time can make a difference. First of all, you should determine if the injury is life-threatening. Immediate recognition of a serious injury can make the difference between life and death or between paralysis and full function. Furthermore, early evaluation is critical in preventing further injury. We all know people who want to play through pain. In many cases—but not all—staying in the game will not result in further injury. However, if you evaluate the injury immediately, your assessment may be more accurate. If you wait, pain, swelling, and muscle spasms may occur. These are natural responses to injury, but they can make evaluation difficult, even for trained medical professionals. Injuries are easier to identify before the entire area becomes swollen or too sore.

Early evaluation may give you more treatment options. For example, let's say your daughter injures her ankle in a volleyball game one afternoon. If you evaluate your daughter's injury when it occurs, you can decide whether to take her to a physician or allow her to rest. However, if you don't evaluate the injury until several hours later, after the ankle has swollen, you may not be able to tell how serious it really is. An unnecessary trip to the emergency room for a minor ankle sprain can turn out to be costly and time consuming.

Performing an Injury Evaluation

The key to evaluating any injury is to be thorough and systematic. This means that you should do the same things every time you evaluate an injury. Using this approach makes injury evaluation routine and reduces the likelihood that you will forget anything. Physicians, nurses, athletic trainers, and physical therapists all learn systematic approaches to injury evaluation. The following are critical points to remember when evaluating your child's injury.

Remain calm and self-confident. People will react to an injury in many different ways. Some will cry and scream, others will get angry and yell. Almost every injured child is scared. As a coach or parent, being confident and in control reduces everyone's stress level. To calm a crying athlete, have him or her slowly breathe in through the nose and out through the mouth. A calm person will give more accurate information than an upset person.

Be thorough, and handle the injury with extreme care. Missing an important sign or symptom can cause further problems. Never assume the injury is insignificant. One coach said that his injured running back was being a "wimp" and told him to play through the pain. When the athletic trainer evaluated the injury later, she discovered that the athlete had a dislocated shoulder! The coach should have taken a few seconds to observe the injury. If he had seen the deformity, he would have removed the child from play.

Never distort the injury. Injured athletes take every word seriously. Even if the injury looks disgusting, never exaggerate its seriousness. Parents and athletes get very nervous when they assume the worst. They are equally worried if you minimize a serious injury. Be honest, but stay calm.

Be conservative. If you make an error evaluating an injury, always err on the conservative side. No game, practice, or event is more important than a child's future health. Never let the importance of a single game or practice skew rational thinking. Let doctors and athletic trainers be the aggressive ones. It is always better to say, "My child could have played," than to say, "My child should not have played."

Remember that the systematic approach is always best. The first step in any injury evaluation is to assess the ABCs: Airway, Breathing, and Circulation. An injury evaluation is meaningless if the athlete cannot breathe or if his or her heart is not beating. Read the chapter on Emergency Procedures for how to deal with a life-threatening situation.

SPORTS MEDICINE AT A GLANCE

An Injury Evaluation

1. GET A HISTORY
2. LOOK AT THE INJURY
3. TOUCH THE INJURY
4. ASSESS RANGE OF MOTION AND STRENGTH
5. PERFORM FUNCTIONAL TESTS
6. CHECK BLOOD SUPPLY AND SENSATION

Parents and coaches do not need to know every possible way to evaluate injuries. Following these simple steps will help you tremendously in developing your own evaluation plan.

1. Take a history. Get answers to these questions:
   - *When did it happen?*
   - *Where did it happen?*
   - *Where does it hurt?*
   - *Can you point with one finger to the place it hurts?*
   - *What were you doing when it happened?*
   - *How did it happen?*
   - *Have you ever hurt this before?*
   - *Did you hear or feel anything pop, snap, crack, or tear?*

If you witnessed the injury, you may already know the answers to these questions. When athletes say that the injury has worsened over time, the injury is probably a chronic inflammation that does not need urgent care or a visit to the emergency room. When athletes know exactly when it happened and can describe what they felt, the injury may be more serious.

2. Observe the injury. Looking closely at the injury can be critical. Check for swelling, discoloration, or deformity. A broken collarbone,

for example, will often look so deformed that physicians know it is broken before the x-ray. You may need to remove a sock, shoe, or other piece of clothing to look at the injury. How would you know if a toe is swollen or deformed if you do not remove the shoe? You should also compare the injured side with the uninjured side. What might appear deformed may be normal for that person's body.

3. Touch the injury. Touch the area very lightly at first, or in a place you know will not hurt. This reduces the athlete's stress and builds his or her confidence in your evaluation skills. If you gently touch the injury, you may be able to determine which structure or tissue is injured. This also helps determine level or intensity of pain. Intense pain or pain that does not subside could indicate a more serious injury.

4. Assess range of motion and strength. This determines how well the athlete can move the injured body part and whether the area is weakened. Excessively weak or limited motions are red flags that mean the athlete needs to see a physician.

5. Perform functional tests. These tests are simple activities that progress from the very easy to the very difficult. For example, assume the athlete has an ankle injury. Ask the athlete to move the injured ankle slowly. If this is no problem, ask the athlete to stand, walk, and then gently jog. If all of these can be done pain free, ask the athlete to run a "figure eight." If any of these activities cause pain, the athlete needs medical treatment.

6. Assess blood supply and sensation. Nerve or blood-vessel injuries can cause permanent damage and require immediate evaluation by a physician. Any numbness or tingling needs immediate attention. Any wound that spurts blood also requires immediate attention (this indicates an injury to an artery).

How Do You Know if It Is Broken?

One of the most difficult but important parts of injury evaluation is to determine if the athlete has broken, or fractured, a bone. This can be difficult for physicians and athletic trainers as well. Diagnostic tests, such as x-rays, MRIs, and CT scans, are the only way to know. Although people learn in basic first aid to treat all injuries like fractures, fracture injuries have certain characteristics.

The primary symptom of a fracture is pain at the fracture site, focused on the bone. Injuries to soft tissues like muscles and tendons do not hurt as much as injuries to bones. This pain usually remains constant or gets worse with motion, stress, or palpation (touching). The athlete may have heard a grinding sound or felt a crack, snap, or grating sensation. Some fractures cause deformity and immediate swelling. Fractures may also cause black-and-blue marks (called ecchymosis) at the injury.

In all cases, if you suspect a fracture or if you are unsure, splint the area and take the athlete to an emergency facility. Two rolled-up magazines or old towels make a good splint. If you notice severe bleeding or a bone sticking out of the skin, call 911. Do not move the affected body part. Control the bleeding and treat the athlete for shock until the ambulance arrives.

Know the Red Flags

Because injury evaluation can be complex, knowing the red flags—indications of serious problems requiring immediate medical attention—may be your greatest tool. Most of the injuries you see or evaluate will be minor. You will be able to provide immediate care for most wounds (minor scrapes and abrasions) and bruises. However, knowing when to get help for athletes with red flags will guarantee they receive the best possible care.

Some red flags indicating serious injury are:

- Signs of fracture. The athlete needs immediate care (splint, cast) and the doctor may order medication to reduce pain.
- Severe pain.
- Severe bleeding (especially spurting blood). Wounds that continue to bleed may require sutures to keep the wound closed. In addition, the doctors and nurses will want to disinfect the wound to reduce the risk of infection.
- Wounds and injuries to the head or face. Falling off a bike or the playground jungle gym can cause serious head injuries. Concussions can be very serious and need to be evaluated by a physician, especially if the child does not

feel better within a few minutes. Persistent headaches, nausea, ringing in the ears, dizziness, and vomiting are serious red flags!

- Any numbness, tingling, or abnormal weakness. Any of these may indicate a nerve injury, which would require an immediate evaluation.

SPORTS MEDICINE AT A GLANCE

Red Flags: Seek Immediate Treatment

- NO BREATHING
- NO PULSE/CIRCULATION
- WOUNDS THAT SPURT BLOOD
- UNCONSCIOUSNESS
- AMNESIA
- DIZZINESS
- EXTREME HEADACHE
- NAUSEA OR VOMITING
- RADIATING PAIN DOWN ARMS OR LEGS
- NUMBNESS IN ARMS AND LEGS
- SLURRED OR INCOHERENT SPEECH
- HOT, DRY SKIN
- EXTREME PAIN
- BONE DEFORMITY/DISLOCATION/OBVIOUS FRACTURE

Injury Treatment: Heat or Ice?

Ice is the treatment of choice. While an injury may sometimes benefit from heat, immediate care should always include ice. Ice eases pain much like an anesthetic and reduces swelling and inflammation. Ice also reduces muscle spasms by controlling nerve activity.

When you apply ice, always remind the athlete that it will be cold. Many young athletes are surprised when the ice feels cold. Many then feel a burning or stinging sensation, followed by an aching feeling, then numbness. Instruct the athlete to leave the ice on the area for fifteen to twenty minutes.

Heat is acceptable in some cases, but never immediately after an injury. Heat increases circulation, which can also increase initial swelling and inflammation. Have an athlete wait until the swelling goes down before returning to activity. At this point, a good rule of thumb is "Heat before and ice after." Warming up injured muscles and tissues before activity is a good idea, because it prepares the body for exercise and helps promote healing. Icing an injury after an activity reduces the inflammation.

Ice Application

There are several ways to ice an injury, all of which are easy to do at home, practices, and athletic events.

- Ice massage. Fill a Styrofoam cup with water and freeze it. When it is completely frozen, remove the sides of the cup (leaving the bottom on makes it easier to hold). Use the ice cup to massage the injured area in a circular motion. This works quickly to ease sore muscles, "jammed" thumbs, and aching knees. Apply ice massage for seven to ten minutes. Keep a couple of ice cups in the freezer so they are ready when you need them.
- Ice bags or packs. Use your imagination with this. Produce bags from your local grocery store, plastic sandwich bags, and even newspaper bags can hold ice. In a pinch, use a bag of frozen vegetables (peas and corn work especially well). Commercial gel-packs work well, too, but they can be more expensive than other methods. If possible, use crushed ice. It conforms to the skin much better than cubes. Remove the air from the bag if you can. This helps keep the ice closer to the skin. To reduce the chances of frostbite, apply a wet cloth between the ice and the skin. Leave the ice on for fifteen to twenty minutes. If you are icing over a wound, soak a sterile gauze pad in hydrogen peroxide and apply it to the skin under the wet cloth.
- Chemical or breakable ice packs. These work well in first-aid kits. They may be used only once, so frequent use can be costly. Apply these the same way as you would ice bags. To "activate" the bag, simply squeeze the bag until you feel a "pop." This pop is what mixes two chemicals inside the bag. Together, these chemicals lower the temperature of the liquid inside the bag. If used improperly, however, the chemicals may leak. Follow the instructions carefully.
- Ice bath. This works well for contoured areas, like ankles, feet, and hands. Snow, or a bucket of water with ice cubes from

the freezer, will work for this. The temperature of the water should be between 50°F and 60°F. Injured body parts need only seven to ten minutes in the bath. Ice baths are especially good for sprained ankles.

RICE

RICE is an acronym that stands for Rest, Ice, Compression, and Elevation. These can help treat almost any injury, but there are some points to keep in mind.

- Rest does not mean sleep or inactivity. To rest an injury means to stop doing things that cause pain. For example, someone with a foot injury may be able to swim without pain. Someone with a shoulder injury may be able to do light jogging. If your son or daughter has an injury, encourage him or her to do activities that don't cause pain. This is not only beneficial to the injury, it is also good exercise.
- Ice. See page 47.
- Compression means applying light pressure to the injured area. ACE bandages (a brand of elastic bandages found at most drug stores) work very well to compress an injury. In a pinch, women's nylons can also provide compression. Compression wraps are especially helpful in treating injuries like sprained ankles or knees. Remember not to wrap the injury so tightly that circulation is restricted, causing numbness or coldness.
- Elevation. Most people use pillows to elevate a sore knee or ankle. However, if you've tried to sleep this way, you've probably noticed that the pillow often ends up on the floor in the morning. Place a hard-sided suitcase or sturdy dresser drawer under the mattress (don't try this with a waterbed, of course). No matter how the person rolls around at night, the injury will always be elevated.

Prevention of Athletic Injury

Parents, coaches, and the athletes themselves all share responsibility for making sure sports are safe. While injuries will occur regardless of everyone's best efforts, there are some very important and simple ways to prevent many injuries.

Athletic equipment can either prevent or cause injuries. When purchasing sports equipment, parents and coaches must carefully consider cost, protective ability, and effect on performance. Never cut corners on safety to save a couple dollars. Make sure that the equipment does what it is supposed to do. And remember, some protective pads or braces may look impressive, but they may have little actual protective value. Never sacrifice protection for cost or performance.

Protective equipment should protect the athlete under all circumstances. Soft, pliable padding may look like the greatest pad ever produced, but it may not hold up under a hard hit. Furthermore, protective equipment must fit well. This may sound obvious, but not everyone follows this important rule. A kneepad, for example, doesn't do much to protect the knee when it is worn around the lower leg. Poorly-fitted helmets can cause serious injury—even death—for athletes in contact sports such as hockey and football.

Protective equipment must never injure an opponent. This, too, may sound obvious. However, one high-school football player and his father were charged with criminal activity when they sharpened the edges of a helmet snap, causing deep cuts to the boy's opponents.

Some players have a false sense of security when playing with protective padding. It makes them feel invincible. These kids may play without regard for their personal safety or the safety of others. It is important to teach kids to take responsibility for their actions and remind them that padding cannot prevent every injury.

In many sports, protective padding isn't always worn by the athletes. Wrestling mats, gymnastics equipment and floor padding, and football goalpost padding are necessary for the athletes' protection. Naturally, there are precautions that must be taken with this equipment as well. In wrestling, for example, coaches and parents can prevent the spread of infections by disinfecting the mats regularly to reduce fungus and other bacteria.

Each competitive season, parents and coaches should go through the following checklist on protective equipment:

- Thoroughly check all padding, including padding worn by the athletes and padding on the athletic equipment.

- Replace or recondition damaged equipment to meet safety standards. Again, faulty helmets can cause serious injury, even death. A child's life is worth more than the cost of a new football helmet.
- Teach your athletes how to use the equipment properly. Protective padding only goes so far. If athletes play without regard for safety, injuries are likely.
- Inspect the playing surface. Remove all hazards that may cause injury. Look for holes and water sprinkler heads in the field. Wipe water spills from basketball courts. Ice arenas need to have the ice resurfaced often to reduce irregular surfaces, which can also cause injury. It is much better to postpone a game or move to a new location than to risk injury.

Pre-Season Physical

Pre-season physicals are quite common, especially in high-school athletics. Many athletes and parents feel that physicals are a nuisance; however, well-executed physicals can detect injuries and illnesses that may make athletic participation harmful. For example, when Clay, a high-school hockey player, had his pre-season physical, the doctor found a heart defect. Doctors surgically repaired this defect, and he resumed hockey the next season. Had Clay played with this defect, he may have had serious problems.

Pre-season physicals also give important information to coaches and athletic trainers. Medical problems like diabetes and asthma, which can be detected by a physical, can have tragic results if left untreated. However, these problems are quite manageable, and athletes with these diseases compete successfully every day. Wade Wilson, a diabetic, played quarterback in the NFL. Knowing his condition, athletic trainers could prepare for those times when his blood sugar was low.

Pre-season physicals should include a complete orthopedic evaluation. This will reveal any muscle weakness, ligament damage, or other injuries that could cause future problems for an athlete in a specific sport. Knee injuries, for example, may be less trouble for a hockey player than for a soccer player. Physicians, athletic trainers, and physical therapists can make suggestions regarding flexibility and strength training to improve performance and reduce the risk of injury.

Playing Fair

No one wants to see their inexperienced eighty-five-pound son wrestle the one-hundred-and-fifty-pound state champion. Even people in Las Vegas would not bet on this match. Not only would the bigger athlete win, the risk of injury to the younger, lighter athlete would be high. Creating fair competition lowers that risk.

Coaches must consider certain factors when creating a safe and equitable playing field. Whenever possible, match athletes based on skill. Competition between poorly-matched players can result in injury. Besides, athletes who lose every time do not have as much fun. Consider weight and size, especially for contact sports. Try not to match the big kids against the little ones. No child wants to get overpowered every drill. Also consider the emotional maturity of your athletes. One athlete may not be as emotionally prepared for sports as another of the same age. Immature athletes typically do not pay as much attention to proper technique and will approach the game differently than more mature athletes. Coaches and parents need to be prepared to handle this.

Warm-Up and Cool-Down

A proper warm-up and cool-down is essential to help prevent injury and reduce muscle soreness following competition.

An effective warm-up consists of three parts. The first part should be a light jog for five to ten minutes to get the heart and lungs ready for more vigorous activity.

The next part should cover stretching exercises for the major muscle groups. (Ask a doctor or athletic trainer to show you helpful stretches.) Hold each stretch for ten seconds or longer, without bouncing. Bouncing during the stretch is counterproductive because the muscle acts as if it is being pulled apart, not lengthened.

During the third part of the warm-up, athletes should practice drills related to their sport. For example, baseball players will hit and throw, and tennis players will practice serves as well as forehand and backhand shots. This prepares the athlete (both physically and psychologically) for the rest of practice or for the competition.

A cool-down after a game or practice reduces muscle injury and soreness. Encourage players to stretch major muscle groups or even go for a light jog or walk for five to ten minutes. In addition, suggest that players ice sore muscles and joints. You may be surprised how much this helps!

Good Coaches Play It Safe

Every coach or parent should teach his or her athletes the proper way to play safely. For example, football coaches should teach athletes never to tackle with their head down because it could lead to neck and head injuries. Coaches must know the sport and understand how to conduct a safe, yet challenging, practice. Injuries often occur because the coach requires too much from his or her athletes.

Good coaches teach a desire to excel and win, as well as the ability to find victory in defeat. This creates a safe and empowering environment for athletes and parents.

Coaches must understand that they are not only responsible for teaching the sport to young people, but for safeguarding the well-being of the children in their charge. Coaches should have basic first-aid skills and a general knowledge of the injuries common to their sport. Coaches and parents should discuss these issues and develop a clear plan about what to do in emergencies. This is discussed further in the Emergency Procedures chapter.

Properly-conditioned players perform better and have fewer injuries than players who are out of shape. Coaches and parents should encourage conditioning (within reason) to help prevent injury. If injury does occur, well-conditioned athletes of all ages will recover much more quickly than more sedentary individuals.

Contact your local TV or radio station for the weather forecast. High temperature and high humidity can cause heat illness, which can be fatal if untreated. You would never want to place an athlete at risk because of the weather. Weather that is too hot or too cold can be dangerous to both players and spectators. We discuss heat illness in the Emergency Procedures chapter.

Athletes should not be allowed to play before their injuries heal satisfactorily. Returning too quickly after an injury can make the problem worse, prolonging the athlete's recovery period. A physician or athletic trainer can help you decide when an athlete is ready to play. While recovering, athletes should stay in shape through activities that do not irritate the injury. For example, a swimmer with sore shoulders could ride an exercise bike or jog on a treadmill.

Injured athletes may return to competition when:

- The injury is no longer painful.
- The body part has regained full strength and full range of motion.
- The athlete can perform the activities required by the sport.
- The athlete is mentally ready.

First-Aid Kits

All teams need a first-aid kit to prevent injuries from becoming worse. Even a minor blister, for example, can turn into a major injury if it becomes infected. Treating the wound right away can prevent complications.

A well-stocked first-aid kit should contain the following:

- Chemical (breakable) ice packs or plastic bags for ice
- ACE bandages of various sizes
- Triangular bandage (may be used as a sling)
- Regular and butterfly bandages
- Athletic tape of various widths (1", 1-1/2", and 2")
- Pre-wrap
- Tape adherent and tape remover
- Bandage scissors
- Sterile gauze pads
- Steri-strips (to hold wounds closed)
- Foam rubber (for extra padding)
- Insect sting kit
- Non-sterile exam gloves (to reduce the transmission of blood-borne diseases, such as HIV or Hepatitis B)
- Medical waste bag (for bloody towels, bandages, gloves, etc.)
- Hydrogen peroxide

- Antibacterial soap and ointment
- Spare contact-lens case
- Tongue depressors
- Cotton swabs
- Petroleum jelly
- Safety pins
- Mirror
- Penlight
- List of emergency telephone numbers

Conclusion

Knowing the red flags and the basics of injury evaluation is an important duty for parents and coaches of young athletes. Remaining calm and direct will ease everyone's stress. A high-school wrestler injured his airway during a match and had difficulty breathing. A concerned parent raced out of the stands and began screaming for high-tech ER equipment. The athlete did not need these products—he needed to remain calm. Because of a spectator's hysteria, he got scared and his airway went into spasm.

Frequently Asked Questions

Q: *My daughter twisted her ankle. Should I take her to the emergency room?*

A: This depends on the injury. A sprained ankle does not require emergency care (in fact, you may wait a long time to see a doctor at an ER). Sprains (ligament tears) hurt on the soft tissue near the bone, while fractures (broken bones) hurt on the bone itself. Moving the bone away from the fracture site can also cause pain.

Whether your daughter's ankle is broken or sprained, splint the area and apply ice. If the pain is so severe that your daughter can't function normally, go to the emergency room. Otherwise, if she is stable and has no red flags signifying a serious problem, make an appointment for her to see your family doctor as soon as possible.

Q: *If one of my players hurts his foot, should I take his shoe off or leave it on?*

A: Take the shoe off. If you can't see the injury, you have no idea what his foot looks like or how severe the injury is. Applying ice through a shoe doesn't do a whole lot of good, either. Remove the shoe and follow your standard injury evaluation plan.

Q: *I am concerned about the equipment for the youth football program. The helmets never seem to fit the kids. Am I an overprotective parent, or should I say something?*

A: By all means, say something. Scream until someone listens. Football is a rough sport, even when the equipment fits. Proper equipment can prevent many injuries; a good helmet can even save a child's life. Never allow your children to practice or play in substandard equipment.

Q: *My daughter hurt her shoulder earlier this year, and it still hurts when she swims. Is it okay for her to swim in the big meet?*

A: If she has an overuse injury (which is the most common type of shoulder injury for swimmers), she probably won't do more damage to her shoulder if she swims in one meet. Be careful, however, that one meet doesn't turn into two or three or four.

Complete rehabilitation prevents many recurring injuries. Possibly, your daughter started swimming again before her injury had fully healed. A physician or athletic trainer can help you determine when she is ready to swim again.

Contributing Author: Steve Marti, MS, ATC/R

Steve is a certified athletic trainer with the Institute for Athletic Medicine, where he holds administrative responsibilities. He also is the Head Athletic Trainer for Robbinsdale Armstrong High School. He has held both positions for eleven years. Steve has been active in the field of athletic training for over twenty years. He recently received the National Athletic Trainers' Association Service Award for dedicated and outstanding service in the field of athletic training.

Contributing Author: Gary Smith, MEd, ATC/R

Gary is a certified athletic trainer at the Institute for Athletic Medicine, Braemar Clinic, and he is the Head Athletic Trainer at Eden Prairie High School. Gary has held several positions with IAM (he was one of the original IAM employees) over the years. He has also held positions in the National Hockey League, and he was the Head Athletic Trainer for the 1980 Gold Medal Olympic Hockey Team. Gary and his wife, Linda, have three children: Tony, twenty-eight, and twins Becky and Todd, twenty-five.

Chapter

4

Emergency Procedures

Youth sports are generally safe. Coaches know more about athletic injuries than ever before, and athletic trainers provide quality medical care to high-school students throughout the country. Protective equipment has never been better, and weight-training programs in many high schools have helped kids become stronger and less likely to be injured.

However, no matter how hard we try to avoid it, injuries will always be a part of sports. Amy, a high-school hockey player, was checked into the boards head first. When she fell to the ice, she could not move her arms or legs, and she had difficulty breathing. A certified athletic trainer was present and handled the situation properly. Fortunately for Amy, she suffered only a mild strain of the muscles in her neck (and a good scare). Her injuries were treated and she was playing hockey again in less than a week.

Circumstances may have been different without an athletic trainer at the game. Imagine your reaction as a parent in a similar situation. How would you feel if no one at the game knew how to handle the problem? Being able to recognize emergencies and develop an emergency plan can literally mean the difference between life and death.

Emergency Plan

This is perhaps the most overlooked part of any sports program. Just as your son practices throwing a football and your daughter practices kicking a soccer ball, parents and coaches should practice their emergency plan.

Develop this plan before the season starts. Waiting until after a serious injury happens is negligent and doesn't help the child who is hurt. Handling a stressful situation without a plan of action is difficult, especially when a child's life is at risk. Practicing the emergency plan and being prepared to act can save precious time when it counts the most.

At least one person at all events, especially contact sports like football and wrestling, should have current CPR certification. Ideally, the certified person should be the coach, but it could also be a member of the team. Make sure to update this certification every year.

Coaches, players, and parents need access to a telephone. If 911 is not supported in your area, make sure that everyone knows the local number for emergency medical systems (EMS) and record this number in your first-aid kit. Always keep small change—enough for a nearby pay phone—in your first-aid kit, in case you need to make an emergency call. If your school district or organization has access to a cellular telephone, that is even better.

Know the easiest route for EMS to the playing area. Simply telling the 911 operator that you are playing at the high school does not save time. In fact, paramedics may waste a minute or two finding your location. Instead, give the operator precise directions, like "We are at the northwest field behind the high school. The second gate will be open for the ambulance."

Designate one person—preferably someone who can remain calm under pressure—to make any emergency calls. Also designate an alternate person in case the first person is not available. The caller should be able to give a brief description of the emergency situation, including the exact location, the number of injured people, the extent of their injuries (if possible), and any first aid that is being given. This information helps the paramedics tremendously.

Distribute the emergency plan to everyone involved with the team, including parents, coaches, athletes, and school officials. This plan will clearly identify who is responsible for specific tasks and will guarantee that emergency situations will be handled efficiently.

All coaches should have up-to-date information about what to do for each athlete if he or she is injured. Johnny, for example, may need to go to Hospital A, while Susie's mother would like her daughter sent to Hospital B. In today's managed-care health system, insurance regulations make this even more important.

Prepare for a wide range of emergencies. Not only should you be able to handle a neck injury, you should also think about what to do in cases of heat stroke and diabetic reactions. Make sure your plan covers all possible situations.

If you need to use your emergency plan, stay calm.
Be prepared to tell the paramedics the following:

1. What happened. Like all medical professionals, emergency personnel find this basic information valuable.
2. The treatment given. If you administered any type of medication because you thought it would help, tell the paramedics. They need to know everything about this athlete.
3. Whether the child has asthma, diabetes, or allergies to medications. The paramedics will relay this information to the emergency-room physicians.

Your emergency plan will protect the athletes in your care and help them get the treatment they need. Having a plan in place also demonstrates a reasonable concern for your athletes, should anyone raise liability questions about your actions. In today's litigious society, this is a good risk-management strategy for coaches and program directors.

The Pre-Evaluation Procedure

Assume you are the coach of a high-school soccer team, and your goalie is kicked in the head and falls to the ground. It is your job to assess the situation. Before you can help the athlete, you need to evaluate and take control of the environment. There are several concerns to keep in mind.

Make sure there is no immediate danger to you or the injured athlete before you try to help. While this may seem obvious, it is easy to leap to someone's rescue without assessing the situation first. Matt, a student athletic trainer, wanted to help an injured hockey player before the play had been whistled. As he ran onto the ice, another hockey player took a slap shot that almost struck Matt in the head. Matt failed to think of his safety when trying to help the injured athlete. Remember, you are no help to the injured athlete if you get injured in the process. If the athlete is still in danger, do what you can to help without endangering yourself.

On your way to the injured athlete, think about what the problem may be. If the athlete is holding his or her ankle, you can probably guess that he or she has an ankle injury. On the other hand, an athlete who lies on the ground without moving could be seriously hurt.

Firmly request that other people, including team members and parents, stay away from the injured athlete. Too many people can make the situation more stressful for you and the athlete. In addition, crowds of people make it difficult for emergency personnel to reach you.

Never move the athlete until you are certain that he or she does not have a serious neck or head injury. Moving the athlete may cause more damage. If the athlete is wearing a helmet, leave the helmet on. Although you may be trying to help the athlete, removing the helmet can cause serious neck injury. The helmet provides a great base to stabilize the head and neck. You may remove the the facemask by cutting the plastic clips that secure the mask to the helmet. Simple garden shears work very well for this.

Once you reach the athlete, determine if he or she is conscious, unconscious, or somewhere in between. Conscious athletes are alert and able to tell you where they are and what the date is. Most athletes injured in youth athletics remain conscious. If the athlete is unaware of time and place and appears drowsy, but responds when spoken to, the athlete needs medical attention. An unconscious athlete appears to be asleep, but may react to pain. Pinch the athlete's skin while stabilizing his or her head (always assume that a head injury could exist). The injured person may respond by waking up and becoming more alert, or he or she may only wince. If an athlete does not wake up to painful stimulus and does not respond when spoken to, this is obviously a medical emergency.

Primary Survey

The primary survey is critical in serious athletic injuries. During this survey, you'll check the injured athlete's airway, breathing, and circulation—the ABCs. Ultimately, the health and safety of your child or athlete depends on the decisions you make in this survey.

Maintaining an open airway is your first concern in all emergency situations. Athletes will never die from a broken arm, but they will die if their airway closes. In addition, an open airway is necessary for mouth-to-mouth resuscitation to be successful.

Listen for the sounds of breathing. Because football and hockey players wear a lot of protective padding, you may not notice a person's chest rise and fall, but you may be able to hear the person breathing. In ice hockey, you may even see the warm breath in the cold arena. If the athlete is on his or her stomach, place a hand mirror near the person's nose or mouth. If the athlete is breathing, the mirror will fog over. If the athlete is on his or her back, you might put your hand or cheek by the person's mouth to feel for breathing.

Listen for abnormal sounds like wheezing or gasping, and determine if the breathing is shallow or deep. Shallow breathing happens when the person does not fully inhale, like when you take a short, quick breath. Deep breaths happen when someone takes a full breath in. If a person has shallow breaths and appears to gasp for air, contact 911 immediately.

If the athlete is not breathing, you must try to open the airway. For young athletes, the most common cause of a blocked airway is when the tongue falls back in the throat. To open the airway, use either the jaw-thrust method or the head-tilt, chin-lift method.

Use the jaw-thrust method if you suspect a head or neck injury. This method does not move the neck at all. Place your thumbs behind the athlete's jaw, with your fingers on his or her cheeks.

Use your thumbs to thrust the jaw forward. Look, listen, and feel for five seconds. This may open the airway enough to allow air to pass through.

Use the head-tilt, chin-lift method only if you are certain the athlete does not have a head or neck injury. Place the heel of one hand on the athlete's head, then place two or three fingers of the other hand on the athlete's chin. As you tilt the head with one hand, lift the jaw with the other. If a person is unconscious, you will be able to tilt the head back quite far. Do not worry—this is normal and may help the athlete breathe. Look, listen, and feel for breathing for five seconds. Again, only use this method if you do not suspect a neck injury.

If the athlete does not begin breathing on his or her own, even after you have opened the airway, you will need to begin mouth-to-mouth resuscitation. Basic first-aid and CPR classes teach this procedure very well. Everyone, especially coaches, should take these courses. You never know when you may need to provide assistance. Contact your local fire department or American Red Cross for information regarding first-aid and CPR classes.

If the athlete is breathing, you will want to check circulation. Knowing the speed and strength of the heartbeat will help medical personnel. If the athlete's heart is not pumping, you will need to do chest compressions. Both the American Red Cross and American Heart Association teach courses in this that every parent should take. Obviously, any person who does not have a heartbeat requires advanced life support. Contact 911 immediately.

Secondary Survey

Assuming the athlete has normal ABCs, you are now ready to evaluate the injury. In the secondary survey, you will find normal or abnormal signs and symptoms of injury. As a parent or coach, your job is not to determine the extent of the injury, but to determine which injuries require immediate attention. In other words, you are looking for red flags.

The following red flags require immediate medical attention:

- Unconsciousness for any length of time.
- Amnesia, ringing in the ears, dizziness, or extreme headache. (These are all signs of possible brain injury.)
- Pupils that are dilated, unequal, or unresponsive to light.
- Memory loss, confusion, or disorientation. (This is not the same kind of confused look your young child gives you when you ask him or her to take out the trash, either!)
- Slow heart rate, low blood pressure, or weak or rapid pulse.
- No pulse. (Begin CPR immediately.)
- Fainting or dizziness.
- Profuse bleeding.
- Shock. (See page 66.)
- Skin temperature that is abnormally hot or cold.
- Abnormal respiratory signs, like shallow or labored breathing.
- Obvious deformity of the bones or joints.
- Clear fluid coming from the ears or nose, which could indicate possible skull fracture.
- Black eyes (which may look like “raccoon eyes”) or bruising behind the ears when the athlete was not hit in the face.
- Skull depressions.
- Blood in the urine or stool.
- Radiating pain in the left shoulder or back (possible cardiac condition).

If you find any of these signs, get medical attention immediately. These can be symptoms of a serious injury or illness.

Shock

Shock is when the body shuts down circulation to save blood for important internal organs, like the brain, liver, and heart. Shock is a natural response to an injury, but it is also an emergency. If you suspect an athlete is in shock, contact 911 immediately. Shock can lead to death if it is not properly treated.

There are several conditions that may cause an athlete to go into shock, including blood loss, severe allergic reaction, sudden drop in blood pressure, and airway obstruction (like when a person chokes on food or injures his or her windpipe). Excessive internal injuries, external bleeding, broken bones, or reactions to medication can also cause shock.

Look for the following signs if you suspect shock in an injured athlete:

- Weak, rapid pulse.
- Cold, clammy skin.
- Nausea, vomiting.
- Itching or burning of the skin.
- Excessive anxiety.
- Loss of consciousness.

If you suspect shock in an injured athlete, first call 911. After you contact 911, do the following:

1. Lay the person on his or her back, with the feet and legs elevated. Only do this if you do not suspect a neck, back, or head injury.
2. Loosen tight clothing.
3. Cover the person to maintain body temperature. If the athlete is a victim of heat illness, however, treat for shock, but DO NOT cover his or her body with blankets. The patient's body temperature is already too high. (See the section on heat illness on page 71 for more information.)

4. Remain calm and reassuring. Too much excitement can cause more problems than the situation itself. Use a soothing voice to calm the athlete.

Head Injuries

Although head injuries are common in contact sports like football, hockey, and wrestling, they can happen anywhere. Your son could fall and hit his head playing basketball, or your daughter could jump for a soccer ball and bang heads with her opponent.

Brain injuries can occur when something strikes the head or when the head strikes an object. When a baseball player takes a ball in the head, for example, the brain may be damaged in the area where the ball made contact. If you were to fall and hit your head, the brain may be damaged on the opposite side when it "bounced" off the inside of the skull.

Head injuries can range from mild to severe. A Grade-I concussion is very mild, and the athlete does not lose consciousness. A Grade-II concussion may involve a brief period of unconsciousness and some degree of amnesia (loss of memory). A Grade-III concussion is the most severe and is accompanied by complete unconsciousness.

Football players are hit in the head often. You may have heard this described as "getting your bell rung." This is a minor head injury. The athletes maintain full consciousness and can remember everything. Aside from a temporary headache, they have no other symptoms. Once this headache goes away (and does not return with activity or exertion), these athletes can safely resume their activity.

Severe head injuries may require surgery. Athletes suffering a Grade-II or -III concussion should not return to activity without a doctor's permission. In most cases, this means at least a week of rest. In some cases, it can be several weeks to months before the athlete may safely return to athletics.

Watch for these red flags with head injuries:

- Headaches that do not improve over a short period of time. Any headache that becomes worse over several minutes requires immediate medical attention. Contact an urgent care center or emergency room as soon as possible.

- Dizziness. Report this immediately, especially if these symptoms do not go away after a few minutes.
- Ringing in the ears.
- Blurred vision.
- Amnesia (the inability to remember events). Some athletes may not remember events before or after the injury. To assess memory, ask athletes questions that you already know the answer to, such as what time practice began or where they are playing. Note, however, that some athletes will try to fool you, especially if they have been through this before. If they cannot answer the questions correctly, seek immediate medical attention.
- Clear, straw-colored fluid (cerebral spinal fluid) coming from the nose or ears. If you see this fluid, contact 911 immediately. Also look for blood coming from the ears or from visible wounds on the head.
- Seizures. In case of a seizure, remove any objects that could injure the athlete. This includes people, benches, equipment, and anything else that the athlete could hit during the episode. It is best to let the athlete come out of the seizure naturally.

Check the athlete's ABCs. If the athlete is unconscious, do the following:

1. Call 911 or your local ambulance service.
2. Treat the athlete with mouth-to-mouth or CPR, if necessary. If you must move the athlete to do this, roll the athlete as one unit while stabilizing the head and neck. (See the following section on spinal cord injuries.)
3. Stabilize the head and neck. To do this, place your hands on the athlete's shoulders, with your forearms on either side of the athlete's head. Rolled bath towels also work well for this. Assume that anyone with a head injury also has a neck injury. (See the following section on spinal cord injuries.)
4. Treat for shock.

Spinal Cord Injuries

Spinal cord injuries can cause paralysis and even death, so it is important to be extremely careful if you suspect this sort of injury. Certain areas of the spinal cord (near the head) carry the information that tells our heart to pump and our lungs to breathe. If this tissue is damaged, the body will no longer get the commands it needs to stay alive. Other areas of the spinal cord (in the middle of the neck) tell our muscles to work. If this area is damaged, we lose the ability to move our arms or legs, for example.

Not all spinal cord problems are the result of an accident. Mike, a high-school football player, had burning and tingling sensations going down his neck and into his arms and hands, sometimes several times during each practice or game. Thinking the problem was insignificant, Mike put up with the discomfort for a year before he mentioned it to the team's athletic trainer. The athletic trainer sent Mike to a physician. After examining Mike, the doctor ordered CT and MRI scans (diagnostic tests, like x-rays). The results showed that Mike was missing a portion of a cervical vertebra in his neck, which protects the spinal cord. This wasn't a life-threatening problem, but it increased his chances of serious spinal cord injury. Mike ended up quitting football—the risk was just too great. Because of the athletic trainer's concern and the doctor's skill in identifying this condition, Mike avoided a serious, perhaps paralyzing, injury.

Although severe back and neck injuries are very rare, every parent and coach should know what to look for and what to do in case of a back or neck injury. Look for:

- Pain on or near the spine. The tiny bumps on the spine are portions of the vertebrae that protect the spinal cord. Injury to these bones can indicate possible damage to the spinal cord.

- Numbness, tingling, or burning or radiating pain in the arms, fingers, hands, toes, legs, or feet. The tingling sensation feels as if the area is "asleep."

- Weakness or inability to move arms, legs, fingers, or toes.

- Deformity. You may notice that the neck is bent at an odd angle, or you may feel the deformity when you gently touch the area.
- Breathing problems.
- Loss of bladder or bowel control. Nerve signals control these functions as well.

If you see any of these signs or symptoms, you need to act quickly. Do the following:

1. Call 911. Trained medical personnel must handle these situations.
2. Do NOT move the athlete unless it is absolutely necessary. You might need to move the athlete to safety (removing an injured diver from the pool, for example) or roll a person over to begin mouth-to-mouth resuscitation. In both cases, you must know exactly how to perform these maneuvers to avoid complicating or worsening the injury. If you do need to move the athlete, always stabilize the head and neck and roll the body over as one unit. Avoid moving the neck at all.
3. Stabilize the head and neck, preventing the athlete from moving and causing further injury.
4. Check the ABCs. Begin mouth-to-mouth resuscitation if necessary. Again, if you absolutely must move the athlete to do this, stabilize the head and neck and roll the athlete's body as one unit. Provide CPR if necessary. If needed, use the jaw-thrust method to provide mouth-to-mouth resuscitation.
5. Provide reassuring support to the athlete.
6. Control the crowd. Several people often gather around the injured athlete, most of whom cannot help. Encourage others to give the athlete "room to breathe." This reduces the athlete's stress and fear as well.

Knowing what to do in these situations can prevent further damage. In fact, your actions may save the athlete's life.

Heat Illnesses

While anyone can have a heat-related illness, young children and elderly adults are at particular risk. For athletes, practicing in hot summer weather can be dangerous. This is especially true for football players and soccer players who practice in early August. When the temperature and humidity are high, parents and coaches must provide opportunities for their children or athletes to cool down.

Heat cramps, heat exhaustion, and heat stroke are the three types of heat illnesses. Heat cramps are signals to stop activity and cool down. Heat exhaustion can be dangerous if untreated. Heat stroke is a medical emergency.

Heat cramps are painful muscle spasms that occur during exercise. These are much like the cramps that might wake you up in the middle of the night. They can appear anywhere on the body, although most occur in the hamstrings, quadriceps, calves, and abdominal muscles.

No one knows exactly what causes these cramps, although experts do have a few possible explanations. Cramps can happen when the body loses important electrolytes (salts that regulate muscle contractions) through sweat. The loss of electrolytes is related to water loss. Cramps can often be prevented it the athlete drinks plenty of water throughout the day, especially during activity, and maintains a balanced diet. Encourage athletes to eat a slice or two of fruit during half-time to replenish electrolytes that may have been lost during the game or practice.

Although a heat cramp is extremely painful, the treatment is simple. First, ask the athlete to sit down. This reduces the stress to the muscle. Then, gently massage or stretch the cramped muscle. Give the athlete water. Products like Gatorade and other sports drinks are helpful, but water will work just fine. Have the athlete drink until he or she feels full, then ask that he or she slowly drink some more. The athlete can play again when the cramps are gone.

Heat exhaustion is another common hot-weather affliction for athletes. We sweat to cool our bodies. When sweat evaporates, it releases body heat into the air. Athletes playing in the sun (especially in football gear) will sweat heavily, but they won't feel any cooler, because the sweat is not evaporating quickly enough. If the humidity is high, sweat evaporates even more slowly. Because the body is still hot, it will keep sweating in an attempt to cool itself. Heat exhaustion occurs when the body has lost too much fluid.

Look for the following symptoms of heat exhaustion:

- Dizziness. The pupils may also be dilated.
- Weakness.
- Nausea.
- Headache.
- Cool, clammy skin. The face may look gray or drained of blood.
- Profuse sweating. The athlete's T-shirt will be saturated with sweat.

Do the following:

1. Remove the athlete from the heat. Find a shady spot to rest or bring the athlete inside to an air-conditioned building.
2. Loosen tight clothing and remove equipment to expose the skin to air. (This is especially important for overheated football players.)
3. Provide water and encourage the athlete to drink.
4. Ice the back or neck to help speed cooling. A word of caution, however: Packing the athlete in ice could cool the body too quickly.
5. Call an ambulance if symptoms do not improve or if they worsen.
6. Anyone with heat exhaustion should spend the rest of the day resting, out of the heat.

Heat stroke is a life-threatening condition that occurs mostly during hot, humid weather. Heat stroke happens when the body's cooling system shuts down completely in order to retain the fluids that the organs need to function. The body stops sweating, and, as you might expect, it overheats, much like your car does without radiator fluid.

Look for the following signs of heat stroke:

- Red, hot, dry skin. This would indicate that the sweating mechanism has stopped. (Cold, clammy skin, on the other hand, is a sign of heat exhaustion.)
- High body temperature. Some athletes with heat stroke have had temperatures over 105°F.
- Unconsciousness.
- Rapid pulse. Because the body is low on fluids, the heart must pump extra fast to get blood to the tissues.
- Vomiting.
- Seizures.
- The heart or lungs might stop working (called cardiac or respiratory arrest) in severe heat stroke cases. Obviously, this requires immediate treatment.

To treat heat stroke, do the following:

1. Determine if the athlete is conscious (if the athlete is unconscious, monitor ABCs—see page 63).
2. Contact 911. The athlete needs fluids, probably delivered intravenously.
3. If the athlete is conscious, move the athlete to a cool area, like a locker room. (Never move an unconscious athlete. Wait for the paramedics to arrive, instead.)
4. Remove all the athlete's clothing and equipment. These will only interfere with the body's cooling system.
5. Use cool water or cool, wet towels to lower the athlete's body temperature. Do not put the athlete in a cold shower. You could induce hypothermia (see page 74).
6. Monitor the ABCs.
7. If the athlete is conscious, have him or her suck on ice chips or take small sips of cool water.
8. Never allow the athlete to return to athletics until cleared by a physician.

There are logical precautions you can take as a parent or coach to prevent heat-related illnesses from occurring. Avoid practicing in high heat and humidity. Always provide several rest and water breaks during practice. Encourage athletes to drink fluids before and after each practice or game. If possible, provide a hose to spray athletes when they become too hot. This is especially helpful for football linemen or hockey goalies, who wear a lot of protective padding. Keep an eye on larger athletes, who are more susceptible to heat illnesses because of their greater body mass.

Cold-Related Injuries

Injuries due to cold exposure are most common in sports like skating, skiing, and ice hockey. Typically, cold injuries (like frostbite) are not life-threatening, but they can be serious if untreated. White or grayish skin is a sign of first-degree frostbite. Contact a physician immediately if the skin is numb or blistered (signs of second- or third-degree frostbite).

Hypothermia is another concern. Hypothermia is a life-threatening condition in which the core body temperature falls below 95°F.

Look for the following red flags of hypothermia:

- Itching, burning, or painful skin.
- Numbness or tingling in the extremities.
- Confusion.
- Excessive shivering.
- Muscle stiffness.
- Drowsiness.

If you suspect an injury from cold exposure, remove the athlete from the conditions. Remove cold, wet clothing and wrap the athlete in warm blankets. Be careful not to expose the skin to excessive heat, especially if the person has lost feeling in the area. A person may burn himself or herself because he or she cannot feel when the tissue is hot. You may also give the athlete warm fluids.

Internal Organ Injuries

Because of protective padding, internal injuries are not common in sports today. When they do occur, however, they can be very serious. Internal injuries affect organs like the kidneys and the spleen. Most of these injuries occur in contact sports like hockey, wrestling, and football.

An athlete with an internal injury can go into shock because of blood loss. If your child was struck in the abdomen or kidney area, you will want to monitor him or her closely. Many of these injuries appear normal for several hours after the injury and only become worse later. Once you notice the red flags, contact a physician immediately.

The spleen is located in the upper-left part of the abdomen. The ribs protect it, but blunt force—from a hard tackle or an errant baseball—can cause serious damage. The spleen is filled with blood and blood vessels. The only way to control the bleeding is to remove the organ.

Watch for the following signs of spleen damage:

- Pain in the upper-left part of the abdomen.
- Pain referred to the left shoulder and neck. This is called Kehr's Sign.
- Nausea and/or dizziness.
- Excessive anxiety. The athlete may feel as though there is something tragically wrong.
- Bruising and/or pain at the injury.
- Increased heart rate and rapid, shallow breathing.
- Shock.

Do the following:

1. Call 911 immediately.
2. Place the athlete comfortably on his or her back. Also, turn the head to the side in case of vomiting. This prevents choking.

3. Treat for shock. Monitor ABCs and provide CPR or mouth-to-mouth resuscitation, if necessary.

A bruised kidney results from a direct blow to either side of the mid back. This can occur when a football player's helmet strikes another player from behind or when a soccer player falls to the ground and is kicked by an opponent.

Look for the following signs of a bruised kidney:

- Pain at the injury. This pain may be located at the front of the abdomen or groin region.
- Nausea or vomiting.
- Blood in the urine. Urination may also be painful.

If you suspect a kidney injury, contact your physician immediately. In all cases, treat for shock and monitor the athlete's condition.

A person can also bruise or lacerate (cut) the liver. The liver is a large internal organ that is filled with blood. The ribs protect the liver, but blunt forces can cause injury. Many of the symptoms are the same as spleen injury; however, the pain is located more on the upper-right side of the body than the left. Suspected injuries to the liver need medical attention immediately.

Appendix injuries are not typically caused by athletics, and appendicitis is not considered an athletic injury. However, appendicitis is not uncommon among school-age children. Although the appendix has no known function, appendicitis causes prolonged and sometimes excessive pain in the lower-right part of the abdomen. If your child suffers from these symptoms, consult your physician.

Conclusion

Sports are great for children. Being on an athletic team encourages teamwork, cooperation, and competition. Participation encourages physical fitness and leads to good habits later in life. However, your child risks injury when playing. We cannot shield children from all injuries, most of which will be minor.

But knowing what to do in those rare exceptions can mean life or death for your child or player.

Always allow trained medical professionals to handle the situation. Physicians, athletic trainers, and paramedics are the most qualified to treat serious injuries. They are trained to respond to life-threatening situations. If your local high school does not have an athletic trainer, encourage your school administrators to provide this valuable service.

Require that all coaches be certified in CPR and first aid. While the emergencies covered in this chapter may never happen, coaches—and parents—should be prepared in case they do. Besides, coaches may be liable if they do not provide immediate first aid. Many legal experts will agree that parents can reasonably expect coaches to understand CPR and first aid. By not having these skills, coaches risk liability.

Finally, know your red flags. Always contact 911 if you suspect a head or neck injury. No parent wants to say, "I wish we had called. This injury was serious." It is always better to say, "I am glad we called and it was a minor injury."

Contributing Author: Rob Lindsey, ATC/R

Rob is a certified athletic trainer, treating patients and athletes in the western Minneapolis suburbs. In the past, he has worked for the Institute for Athletic Medicine and served as the Head Athletic Trainer for Richfield High School.

Contributing Author: Scott Kulstad, MEd, ATC/R

With Appreciation: Scott Gardner, ATC/R

Chapter

5

Issues for Girls and Women Only

We consider this to be one of the most beneficial chapters in this book. We discuss issues that not many people want to talk about, such as eating disorders, osteoporosis, amenorrhea, and stress incontinence—all problems that affect mostly girls and women. While we will be the first to say that eating disorders can affect both boys and girls, it is a predominantly female issue. Osteoporosis does not affect males like it does females, and amenorrhea is an exclusively female concern.

Stress incontinence refers to the involuntary loss or leakage of urine. This problem is much more common among adolescent female athletes than people will admit. We hope that parents, coaches, and teachers will not avoid this chapter simply because it addresses concerns that are not fodder for the dinner table.

The issues in the chapter can have a profound impact on a girl's athletic performance and her life in general. Problems left untreated create problems later in life. As an example, one of our therapists is treating a young woman for stress incontinence—every time she runs, she leaks urine. This not only affected her exercise pattern, it kept her from going to dances and socializing with her friends. This young woman waited only several months before mentioning the problem to her doctor, and her treatment has been very successful. However, many people wait an alarming seven to nine years before they tell their physicians. While incontinence is not an easy topic to discuss, we want parents to make a point of asking their daughters about it if they have reason to be concerned. The same is true for menstrual cycles.

Another topic we address briefly in this chapter is pregnancy and exercise. While pregnancy is uncommon among young female athletes, it has been known to occur. Parents and coaches of pregnant athletes should learn how to protect the health of both mother and baby. Furthermore, we have met more than one expectant "soccer mom" who still coaches her ten-year-old daughter's team. Information about pregnancy and exercise will benefit athletes like these as well.

We address female-specific injuries and injury prevention in the Anatomy and Physiology chapter. Specific nutritional concerns for female athletes are discussed in the Exercise, Conditioning, and Nutrition chapter.

We have named this chapter after the program in our clinic system—the For Women Only program—that specializes in the treatment of females (both athletes and non-athletes). When we started this program in 1995, we had only 350 patient-visits in the first year. We expect that our therapists will have over 3,000 patient visits in 1998, and well over 5,000 by the year 2000.

We have made every effort to simplify complex terminology in this chapter. We hope to address the issues with the compassion and sincerity that our patients receive from us daily. Furthermore, we hope that this chapter enables you to talk about these issues, as sensitive as they may be, with the young women you care so much about.

Eating Disorders and Disordered Eating

Young adolescent girls are at a particularly high risk for developing eating disorders. There are many different reasons for this. If you look near the checkout register at your local convenience store, you'll probably see a number of glossy fashion magazines picturing attractive models with skimpy clothing and little body fat. Feature articles in these magazines claim to offer surefire methods for losing weight. Now think about television. Thin models tout fat-free products on commercials, and rarely, if ever, will you see an overweight or heavy actor on

Melrose Place or *Beverly Hills 90210*. Messages from the media teach our children that to look good is to be thin. This places an incredible amount of pressure on children, especially young girls. (In reality, less than 10 percent of the population has the genetic make-up to look like a supermodel.)

This issue can be particularly difficult for girls in sports. On the one hand, many young female athletes want to be thin. Popularity in school, they feel, depends on being thin and beautiful. On the other hand, coaches and athletic trainers recommend strength training and weight training, because strong athletes perform better and have fewer injuries than weaker athletes. However, as strength increases, so does size. Many young girls feel they must choose between being strong and competitive and being beautiful. This creates an internal struggle: Should they eat enough to be competitive, or should they eat to stay thin? As one young athlete said, "I'll eat to stay in my size-four pants."

Luckily, there are many female athlete role models today who are both strong and beautiful. Girls who follow their lead will become more confident and self-reliant as they train to become better and stronger athletes.

Not all young female athletes have eating disorders, but girls who have low self-esteem or who suffer from depression are at a higher risk for clinical eating disorders, such as anorexia nervosa and bulimia. Eating disorders are mechanisms to cope with internal or external stresses and emotional problems. In these cases, the underlying problem is rarely about food or the desire to be thin.

For example, one young woman had a serious back injury that left her unable to play the sport she most enjoyed. While she could live a relatively normal life, she was unable to participate in gymnastics. She began to restrict her food intake. She lost weight, rode an exercise bike constantly, and refused to eat more than five grams of fat per day. In fact, she would break an Oreo cookie into fourths and only eat one of the four pieces. Her eating disorder became her coping mechanism—her way of trying to control a situation over which she really had very little control.

Eating disorders can lead to significant injury, illness, and even death. Many physicians will agree that as many as 20 percent of all eating-disorder patients die each year due to their disease.

Anorexia nervosa and bulimia have similar warning signs, but the two disorders are different. A person may suffer from both at the same time, however.

The following are symptoms of anorexia nervosa:

- The young person eats very tiny portions. Sometimes she hides food or refuses to eat, saying she is not hungry.
- The young person avoids fat, sugar, and/or meat. Anorexic patients refuse to eat foods they feel will make them fat. Medically speaking, the body requires fat. As much as 20 to 25 percent of the diet should come from fat.
- The young person has an intense fear of becoming fat. She may have a significantly distorted body image. Many anorexic patients feel fat even when they are obviously slender. These patients refuse to maintain the recommended minimal weight. This fear of being or becoming fat haunts them and does not subside, even with weight loss.
- Perfectionism is a shared trait among many anorexic patients. These young girls usually excel in everything from academics to athletics. They are typically Type A personalities with a lot of self-control.
- The young person is excessive about exercise. Anorexic patients may work out several hours per day. This type of exercise is more than what would be required for success in youth sports. Either the frequency or the duration of exercise can be abnormal. If you have any questions about whether your child overexercises, consult your physician, a counselor, the school nurse, or an athletic trainer in your area.
- Depression and low self-esteem are common among young people with anorexia nervosa. The disorder is really indicative of a larger problem. Issues such as overbearing stress, emotional upheaval, and psychological problems stemming from rape and sexual violence can trigger episodes of anorexia. One athlete was accepted into a major performing arts studio. However, she was unable to handle the stress of being the best dancer in the area. She became

anorexic to cope with that stress. In the end, she felt as though people liked the dancer, not the person. Many young people suffering from anorexia withdraw from family and friends, which seems to compound the problem.

Bulimia patients also use food to control behavior, but the characteristics of a bulimia patient differ slightly.

Consider the following behavioral signs of bulimia:

- Bulimia patients binge and purge. This means that they eat (perhaps normally, perhaps excessively) and then vomit. Many feel so guilty about what they ate (either the type of food or the quantity) that they find relief when they purge the food. In essence, the food they purge is their guilt or shame. Bulimia patients often have poor self-control.
- Many young people with bulimia disappear to the bathroom after meals. This is most likely when they induce vomiting or use laxatives to rid their bodies of the food and calories they have just eaten. One young girl used syrup of Ipecac to induce vomiting. She did this until she was scared that the Ipecac had calories. She got to the point that after vomiting, she felt she had to vomit again to purge the syrup of Ipecac.
- Bulimia patients are typically impulsive. Some experts feel that people who suffer from bulimia are at high risk for drug and alcohol problems.
- Unlike anorexia patients, bulimia patients appear to eat normal quantities of food in public. Anorexia patients tend to pick at food or order non-fat, low-calorie meals.
- Bulimia patients think of their eating as abnormal.

If you suspect your child or a child you coach has an eating disorder, look for these red flags:

- Excessive exercise.
- Loss or absence of menstrual periods. (We will discuss the effects of amenorrhea in the next section.)

- Unhealthy weight loss (more than 15 percent of body weight).
- Fainting, blackouts, or periods of dizziness. This can be the result of dehydration and/or electrolyte imbalances.
- Brittle hair and nails.
- Loss of tooth enamel. When bulimia patients vomit, the acid from the stomach erodes the enamel on the teeth. Enamel loss can be a sign of vomiting.
- Frequent weight changes. A bulimia patient's weight will seem to fluctuate, while an anorexic patient will typically lose weight.
- Low heart rate, blood pressure, and body temperature.
- Sore throat and/or swollen glands. Bulimia patients irritate their throats quite badly when they vomit. An irritated throat can be a red flag, especially if combined with any of the other signs.
- Raw or irritated fingers. This is not always easy to see, but many bulimia patients rub or scrape their fingers on their teeth when they try to induce vomiting. Again, this red flag will help you evaluate other signs and symptoms. Alone, it may not be enough to suggest a bulimia diagnosis.

If you suspect any of these red flags, you must act quickly. If you choose to ignore a sore ankle or a swollen knee, your child probably will not suffer long-term disability. Ignoring an eating disorder, however, can lead to death. Be proactive. Talk to your child about your concerns. Do not be surprised if she denies a problem. This is quite common. It is much easier for her to continue her eating disorder than to face the underlying issues. Explain to her that you are not punishing her, that you will help her find professional treatment, and that she can be well again. Do not treat eating disorders on your own. Treatment must include medical evaluation by a physician, nutritional counselor, or behavioral counselor. Families should attend counseling as well. This can be a terribly difficult process for all family members. Do not expect easy and quick resolution.

Leaving an eating disorder untreated can have far-reaching ramifications. Dehydration and electrolyte deficiency can lead to cardiac arrest. Prolonged episodes of vomiting can rupture the esophagus and tear blood vessels in the throat, which can lead to choking and death. Depression, which accompanies eating disorders, can lead to suicide. For these reasons, seek professional help. It is foolish to think an eating disorder will go away or that you can help the person on your own.

Amenorrhea

Women train to be bigger, stronger, and faster than ever before. Rigorous training routines, however, can disrupt normal menstruation. Until recently, many people considered this insignificant. Even female athletes considered this a respite from the monthly cycle. We now know that amenorrhea affects up to two-thirds of all female athletes and can lead to problems affecting the woman's skeletal framework.

Normal menstrual cycles occur before age sixteen, and most women have between ten and twelve cycles per year. Most women have between twenty-eight and thirty-five days between each cycle, with each cycle lasting three to seven days.

Amenorrhea can take one of two forms: primary and secondary. Primary amenorrhea is the failure of menstruation to begin before the age of sixteen. Most young women get their menstrual periods before age sixteen, and a pediatrician or family physician should evaluate those who have not. Being physically active can delay the start of menstruation. This does not mean that a young female with primary amenorrhea needs to stop participating in athletics, only that a doctor should evaluate the situation.

Secondary amenorrhea is the disruption of normal menstrual cycles for anywhere between three and twelve consecutive cycles. Many adolescents would view this as a pleasant break from the side effects that often accompany menstruation, but the side effects from amenorrhea can be injurious.

Both forms of amenorrhea are related to the hormone estrogen. Nutrition and body weight affect hormonal levels. Amenorrhea can be common among gymnasts and other athletes with low body fat.

As many as 80 percent of amenorrheic runners consume less than the recommended amounts of protein. Typically, they are also on the low end of carbohydrate, calcium, and iron consumption. As athletes decrease calorie consumption and body weight and increase exercise levels or athletic participation, amenorrhea can become a problem. Some experts suggest that when a female's body-fat percentage drops below 12 to 14 percent, normal menstruation could stop. Girls who start highly-competitive exercise programs when they are very young can delay the start of menstruation and increase their chances of developing primary amenorrhea.

For girls and women who exercise excessively, estrogen can decrease to dangerously low levels. One study showed that only 6 percent of the women who ran ten miles or less per week had amenorrhea. Among women who ran sixty miles or more per week, over 40 percent were amenorrheic.

Amenorrhea causes negative changes in bone density. This is related to decreased levels of estrogen, the hormone responsible for menstruation. Bone density refers to the strength of the bone—higher bone density means stronger bones. In women, bone density usually peaks around age thirty. Around age thirty-five, women begin to lose bone density at a rate of 1 to 2 percent per year. This loss of bone density continues throughout life, but really begins to accelerate after menopause, due to the loss of estrogen.

Because amenorrheic athletes have lower levels of estrogen, they may not reach full bone density by age thirty. In fact, bone density levels of a young female gymnast or diver, for example, may be lower than that of some postmenopausal women. A physician once referred a young marathon runner to us for osteoporosis, or "brittle bone disease." She was twenty-five years old and had not menstruated for ten years. Tests indicated that she had the bone density of a seventy-year-old woman.

Clearly, the premature loss of bone density is neither healthy nor advantageous. Amenorrheic athletes are predisposed to stress fractures, and even minimal trauma can cause complete fractures. Young amenorrheic athletes often experience stress fractures in the same places as elderly women diagnosed with osteoporosis—the spine, upper thigh, lower leg, wrist, and upper arm. Osteoporosis is a progressive disease in which the bones degenerate over time. Patients with the disease suffer from a slumped posture and are very susceptible to fractures. Unfortunately, these changes are irreversible.

Once a woman loses bone density, she will not regain it. She can only modify her activities to compensate for the loss. She can do several things to improve the condition, however. The goal in treatment is to regain normal hormonal levels and chemical secretions, triggering normal, regular menstrual cycles.

Amenorrheic young women should improve their eating and nutritional habits. Many amenorrheic women are nutritionally deficient. They often eat too little within a specific food group—or too little altogether. A registered dietitian can assist in correcting nutritional deficiencies. Remember, changing eating patterns can be difficult, especially since there are often societal pressures that affect the eating habits of young people.

The athlete may also need to change her exercise pattern. Reducing the intensity and frequency of exercise will allow the body to devote more energy to physical growth and development.

If your athlete is amenorrheic, consult your family physician or pediatrician as soon as possible. If all other treatments fail, the physician may suggest estrogen replacement medication. This will help restore proper hormonal balance. Many experts agree that the longer an athlete is amenorrheic, the less likely it is that her condition will improve through medication or physical therapy.

Women today face significant pressures when competing in sports. Many young athletes fall victim to the Female Athlete Triad, which is characterized by amenorrhea, anorexia, and decreased bone-density. Ignoring the signs of amenorrhea can create a life-long problem. Be aware—and make your daughter aware—that although questions about her menstrual cycle may seem a bit too personal, there are very real and important reasons for asking.

Pregnancy and Exercise

Although pregnancy is uncommon among adolescent athletes, coaches should be prepared to handle this situation if it arises.

Every female is different, and every pregnancy is different. Therefore, female athletes who become pregnant should always get consent from their OB/GYN, midwife, or family physician before beginning or continuing athletic activity. They might also ask their doctor for a copy of the *Guidelines for Exercise in Pregnancy,* published by the American College of Obstetricians and Gynecologists (ACOG).

In general, women who participate in athletics before their pregnancy can probably continue exercising, although with less intensity and shorter duration. Pregnant women should stop activity when they begin to feel fatigued, and they should never exercise to the point of exhaustion.

ACOG feels that as body weight increases, the safest exercises are non-weight-bearing activities, such as swimming and cycling. Generally, if the athlete has been jogging before her pregnancy, she may continue to jog as long as her doctor says it is okay. Naturally, her intensity and duration should decrease throughout the pregnancy. If the doctor feels that the athlete should not jog, she may be permitted to do walking and low-impact aerobics, instead.

One problem women frequently experience during pregnancy is low back pain. Changes in posture and hormone levels, preexisting back problems, and improper lifting can all contribute to low back pain.

As the uterus enlarges with the growing fetus, the normal curve of the woman's spine changes. The natural curve in the low back, which is called lordosis, increases as the pelvis tilts forward and the mother gains weight. To adjust for this curve and for changes in the body's center of gravity, pregnant women typically lock or hyperextend their knees and lean backward to maintain balance. This posture creates muscle imbalances that overwork some muscle groups and underwork others. Furthermore, the broad ligament that attaches from the uterus to the front of the lumbar spine stretches as the fetus grows. This creates additional stress on the low back.

Ovarian hormones are responsible for changes in the connective tissues—ligaments, tendons, and fascia—throughout the body. Because connective tissues in the joints loosen during pregnancy, the body is more susceptible to injury. A five- to ten-minute warm-up before activity and cool-down after activity is essential to help prevent injury.

Pregnancy can irritate pre-existing back problems. If your athlete has any conditions that could be affected by pregnancy, you will want to consult with a physical therapist, athletic trainer, or another healthcare provider with specialized training in OB/GYN. These specialists can identify causal factors and treat injuries with the entire body—pregnancy and all—in mind.

Because pregnancy stresses the back, even simple activities—housekeeping, gardening, and personal care—can be difficult. Improper lifting techniques (such as bending at the waist to lift a heavy grocery bag or book bag) can cause additional stress and lead to injury.

With vigorous exercise, back problems can become even more painful. If the muscles supporting the spine are weak, some forms of exercise may cause too much stress to the spine. You will want to consult a healthcare provider to assess muscle strength and flexibility and determine what level of physical activity is right for your athlete.

Pregnant athletes should adopt a moderate exercise program that includes strength training to strengthen the buttock, thigh, abdominal, and low back muscles. This will help prevent or reduce low back pain. For more information about strengthening exercises, consult your physician or physical therapist. A trained professional should monitor and modify these exercises as needed throughout the woman's pregnancy.

The athlete should also dedicate time to stretching exercises. Have her gently stretch tight hip and spine muscles, and make sure she stretches with less intensity than she did before her pregnancy.

The athlete's exercise routine should also include balance training. Pregnancy changes a woman's center of gravity and can make even simple tasks seem awkward. Standing on one leg with the eyes open, then with the eyes closed, can improve body awareness and spinal alignment.

Make sure that your athlete pays specific attention to her posture during her exercise routine throughout her pregnancy. She can do this by remembering to lift properly (by bending her knees to get down to the level of the object and by lifting objects close to her body) and by pointing her feet in the direction she is moving. Remind the athlete to breathe out as she lifts.

If your athlete continues to experience low back pain, have her discontinue the activity that causes the pain. This is not always as easy as it sounds, especially if just sitting in class causes pain. If she can limit the offending activity, her back will appreciate it. Use ice on the back to alleviate pain. Also, consider using a low-back support or sacroiliac stabilization belt (SI belt). You should be able to purchase a low-back support at your local pharmacy or department store. These back supports work well for some patients because they help lift up the abdomen and/or stabilize the pelvis, which reduces stress to the low back. The athlete should be fitted with an SI belt by a medical professional. If all else fails, consult a physician. He or she may refer the athlete to a physical therapist who specializes in OB/GYN issues.

Stress Incontinence

If young women feel uncomfortable talking about their menstrual cycles, discussing stress incontinence will be even more difficult. Stress incontinence is the loss of urine during physical activity. Activities causing stress incontinence can range from coughing and sneezing to running, jumping, and high-impact landing activities. Stress incontinence affects females of all ages, especially females with weak pelvic floor muscles. (Pelvic floor muscles support and cradle the bladder.) There is a common misconception that childbirth causes incontinence and that only those women who have given birth can lose control of their bladder. However, over half of all women who experience some form of incontinence have never had children.

One in five women who suffer some degree of urinary leakage change their mode of exercise (from running to swimming, for example). Over half of them wear protective padding. A 1991 study in *Runner's World* estimated that over 75 percent of the 126 female runners surveyed had urinary leakage when running. They had no other problems at any other time. This is not a topic that women feel comfortable discussing. It is embarrassing to discuss losing bladder control, and many women just deal with it, thinking there is nothing they can do about it.

The bladder is the holding tank for urine. It lies behind the pubic bone, which is the bony structure just behind the pubic hair. The bladder receives urine from the kidneys and stores the urine until it fills up. When it is full, the bladder signals us to use the restroom.

The pelvic floor muscles act as doors to prevent urine from leaking out the tube during everyday activity. These muscles run from the pubic bone to the tailbone. During the emptying phase of urination, the bladder contracts and the muscles relax, allowing urine to exit the body. The urine exits through a small tube called the urethra. (This tube is four to six centimeters long.)

If the pelvic floor muscles are weak, leakage may occur during physical activity. This is one of the main reasons behind the problem of stress incontinence. As abdominal pressure increases during physical activity, this pressure bears down on the bladder. Without strong pelvic floor muscles to keep the urine in, pressure can cause urine to exit the body.

Bladder (Weak Pelvic Floor Muscles)

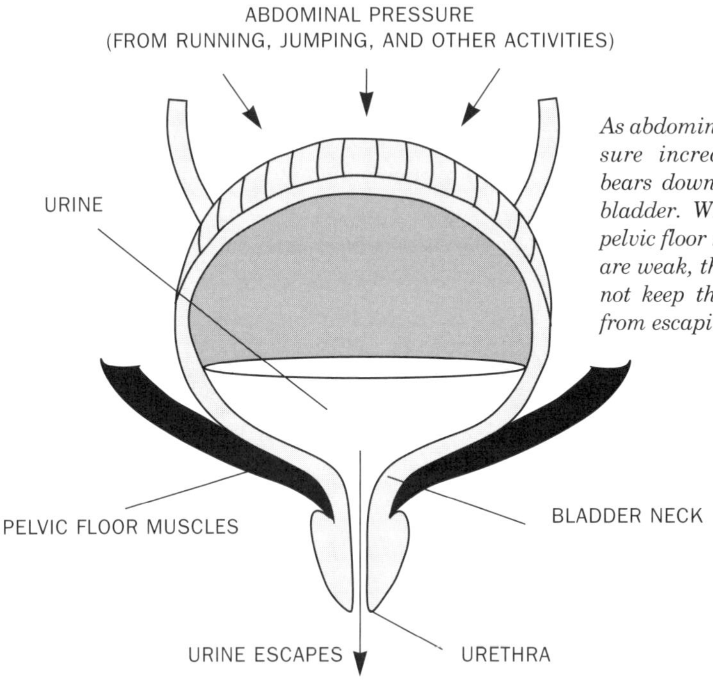

As abdominal pressure increases, it bears down on the bladder. When the pelvic floor muscles are weak, they cannot keep the urine from escaping.

Bladder (Strong Pelvic Floor Muscles)

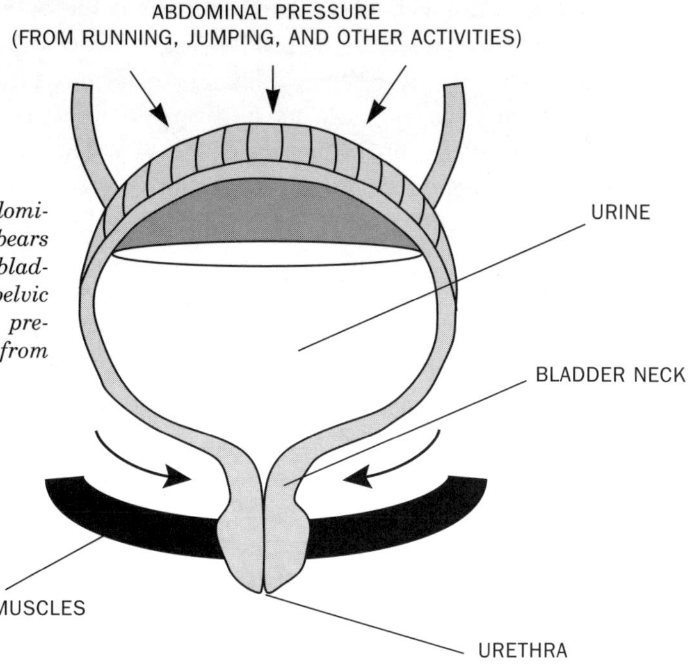

Although abdominal pressure bears down on the bladder, strong pelvic floor muscles prevent urine from escaping.

Physicians and physical therapists who are trained to treat OB/GYN issues can manually assess the strength of a woman's pelvic floor muscles. A woman can also assess her own pelvic floor muscles with the "stop test." Your athlete can perform the stop test next time she uses the bathroom. Ask her to attempt to stop her urine flow midstream. She should be able to stop it abruptly. Failure to stop urine flow could indicate pelvic floor weakness. Your daughter or player should consult a physician if this happens. Do not have your daughter practice this test on a regular basis, as it may disrupt the normal urination process.

One exercise physicians recommend is the Kegel exercise. Because pregnant women frequently experience incontinence when the uterus creates pressure against the bladder, many women learn of this exercise during pregnancy. Some women have difficulty performing this exercise correctly, however. If your young athlete suffers from urinary incontinence, consult a healthcare provider to learn the correct technique for performing this exercise.

There are a variety of treatments for stress incontinence. Diet modification, for example, can help some patients. Some fluids and foods can make the urine very acidic, causing the bladder to try to expel the urine. (If the muscles are weak, it is difficult to hold the urine.) Tomatoes, caffeine, carbonated and alcoholic beverages, tea, acidic foods, and chocolate are examples of bladder irritants. We recommend that people limit bladder irritants and consume fifty to seventy ounces of water per day to dilute the urine—more if they exercise regularly. Diet modification can make strengthening the pelvic floor muscles more effective and more efficient.

Women have heard for years that incontinence is a normal and expected part of being a woman, especially after vaginal births. This is a myth, and many women are learning that exercises and other forms of therapy can reduce or eliminate these periods of incontinence.

Frequently Asked Questions

Q: *The school nurse called me about my daughter. She thinks my daughter is anorexic. I am furious at the nurse for saying that, but I am also worried. What should I do?*

A: Anger and fear are common reactions that parents have when confronting eating disorders. Anorexia is a sign of serious distress, but so few people understand this disease that many people stereotype the disorder and its victims. Make no mistake, you need to see your physician about this. Your daughter needs medical care—the sooner the better.

You should appreciate the nurse's telephone call. Eating disorders kill as many as 20 percent of the people who suffer from them. Failure to seek help is like burying your head in the sand. The problem will not go away on its own—your daughter needs help.

Please do not beat yourself up for feeling angry. Anger is a common response. Learn as much as you can about the disease, and prepare for the marathon. Good luck!

Q: *I have noticed that my sixteen-year-old daughter never asks me to buy her tampons or mini-pads. She must not be menstruating. Is this bad?*

A: Yes. Although they are not life-threatening, the effects of amenorrhea (the absence or cessation of menstruation) are drastic. Amenorrhea can affect bone density, which can lead to osteoporosis. Many people think that osteoporosis only affects elderly women, but this is not true. It is a very serious problem for young people because bone density changes are irreversible. We recommend that you see a physician and perhaps a nutritionist about this.

Q: *I have noticed urine stains on my daughter's underwear after games and practices. She could not be wetting her pants, could she?*

A: Actually, yes, she could. This condition is called stress incontinence and it affects many more young women than people know. Runners and athletes in jumping sports are at risk for this condition. Because the condition is very embarrassing for many people, they often ignore the problem.

Ask your daughter if she has been experiencing any urine leakage. If so, ask your doctor to recommend a physical therapist who specializes in OB/GYN patients. You may be surprised at what a physical therapist can do.

Contributing Author: Heidi Richards, PT

Heidi is a physical therapist with the Institute for Athletic Medicine, Plymouth Clinic, a clinic she also supervises. Heidi treats a variety of sports and orthopedic patients, but she specializes in treating the unique needs of female patients. A member of the IAM For Women Only program, Heidi has helped hundreds of women overcome issues related to pregnancy and osteoporosis. Heidi and her husband, Kevin, have two children, Thomas and Tyler. They live in Brooklyn Park, Minnesota.

Contributing Author: Elizabeth Smith, PT, ATC/R

Elizabeth is a certified athletic trainer and physical therapist with the Institute for Athletic Medicine, Eagan Clinic. Elizabeth is a multi-talented professional. She provides physical therapy to sports and orthopedic patients at the Eagan Clinic, while also being committed to seeing female patients in the IAM For Women Only program. She is also active in the IAM Running Program. Elizabeth and her husband, Kevin, live in Maplewood, Minnesota.

Part Two:

The Details

Chapter 6

Foot, Ankle, Lower Leg, and Toe Injuries

Imagine your daughter telling you she hurt her foot in soccer practice. You may have a hard time assessing what really was injured, especially if you didn't witness the incident that caused the injury. Was it one of the many bones in her foot, her ankle, or one of her toes? Did she injure one of the bones in her lower leg, or did she damage the muscles in her lower leg? This chapter will help you answer some of these questions, offer basic treatment advice, and help you determine the appropriate action.

Anatomy

The anatomy of the foot and lower leg is complex. Three bones—the tibia, fibula, and talus—meet to form the ankle joint. The foot itself has twenty-six bones. Two bones in the lower leg provide support and stability. Twelve different muscles cross the ankle and provide movement to the ankle, foot, and toes.

The tibia is the largest bone in the lower leg. It is a long, thick bone that provides strength and stability when we walk and run. At the ankle joint, the tibia is the bone that produces the large bump on the inside of the ankle. This bump is called the medial malleolus.

The fibula is the smaller bone in the lower leg. This bone is more susceptible to injury from direct trauma (like being kicked) than the much larger tibia. It runs on the outside of the lower leg and creates the bump on the outside of the ankle. This bump is called the lateral malleolus. The fibula serves as a place of attachment for the muscles of the lower leg. Because of its smaller size, it does not provide a lot of stability when we walk and run.

The talus is the bone that fits in between the two bumps to create the ankle joint. The talus rotates forward and back to allow us to point the foot and toes down and to pull the foot back up.

The foot has many small bones that work together to provide stability in our feet when we walk and run. The bones also serve as attachments for the foot muscles that control our movements. The calcaneus is the largest bone in the foot and provides contact with the ground when we walk. We commonly refer to this as the "heel bone." The metatarsals are the long bones between the ankle and the toes. The other small bones in the foot provide stability when the arch of the foot rises or falls when we walk.

Right Foot (viewed from the bottom)

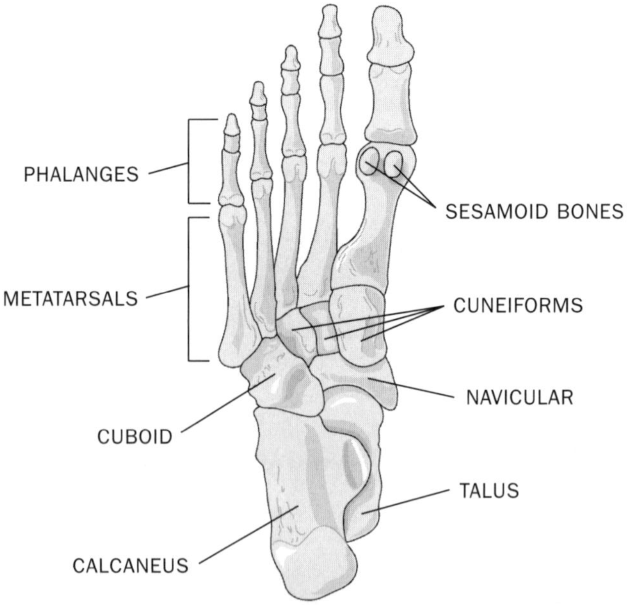

Four compartments divide the muscles of the lower leg. Each compartment holds a group of muscles that perform a specific function, and they all pass through the ankle joint and into the foot to control foot and toe movements. The muscles in the front of the lower leg—held by the anterior compartment—pull the foot and toes up or toward your face. The muscles on the outside—in the lateral compartment—move the outside of your foot up. This causes the bottom of your foot to point away from the opposite foot or leg. The muscles in the deep posterior compartment on the inside of your lower leg do the opposite—they make the inside of the foot turn upward or toward the opposite leg. These muscles raise the arch. The muscles in the back of the lower leg—in the superficial posterior compartment—point your toes and feet down. People use these muscles when trying to stand on their toes. They are very important when we make quick starts and jumps, as we do in basketball, for example.

The muscles in the feet control toe movements. These muscles control activities like curling your toes. As you can see, the anatomy of the foot and lower leg is quite complex. For that reason, evaluating these injuries can be difficult.

Biomechanics

The ankle rotates primarily in two directions—moving the foot upward, or toward the face, and moving the foot downward, or toward the ground. The ankle moves down twice as far as it moves up, which is why you can point your toes and your feet down much farther than you can pull your foot toward your face. The talus—the bone that moves in the ankle joint—fits much more tightly between the tibia and fibula when the foot is pulled up toward the face, resulting in more restricted movement. More ankle injuries occur when the foot is pointing down.

The joints in the foot allow movement, which permits us to tap our feet from side to side. These joints also allow the arch of the foot to become flat or rise high. When the arch falls, we refer to it as pronation. People with excessively pronated feet have "flat" feet. When the arch is high, we refer to it as supination.

The joints in the toes are much like the joints in the fingers. They permit us to move our toes up and down. This movement is critical because the toes need to bend when we walk.

Lower Leg Injuries

Shin Splints

The term "shin splints" refers to any number of disorders in the lower leg. However, most people with classic shin splints have pain three to four inches above the medial malleolus—the inside ankle bone—on the tibia. Your physician may call this medial tibial stress syndrome. Over 80 percent of all shin splint pain occurs in the inside portion of the tibia, although shin splints are not limited to the tibia. Runners and athletes in field sports like football and soccer most commonly suffer from shin splints. Typically, people suffering from shin splints have tendonitis in the posterior tibialis tendon. They may also have inflammation and pain in the soleus muscle and tendon group.

Identifying shin splints is easy, though not foolproof. If you have any questions, please contact your physician. However, before running to the urgent care facility, you may want to think of the following. Shin splints hurt. Although it does not indicate severe injury, a substantial amount of pain is normal. Pain typically is the most severe following competition. Your child will probably not have a lot of pain on the tibia—the bigger bone in the lower leg—but will have a lot of pain just to the side of it.

However, you should keep an eye out for the following red flags. These symptoms indicate a possible stress fracture, which we discuss in the next section:

- Intense bone pain.
- Pain that increases during workouts and is relieved only by rest.
- Any swelling or discoloration in the area.

There are several factors that can contribute to shin splints. One is improper footwear. Some young athletes—and their parents—pay little attention to the shoes they wear during athletics. Some even run in sandals or in old sneakers with holes in the soles. Others wear footwear that is too small or otherwise poorly fitted. Improper footwear does not provide adequate stability for the foot and lower leg.

Athletes who train every day or almost every day need to pay close attention to how often they replace their shoes. For example, we typically recommend that runners change shoes every three hundred to five hundred miles. Many parents may not like to hear, "Hey, Mom and Dad, I need new shoes! It says so here in the book," but new running shoes do make a difference. One patient suffered shin splints for over a year before she saw us for therapy. We recommended that she get new shoes. Within two weeks, her pain was gone.

Another cause of shin splints is a poor running surface. Athletes in northern climates do not have the luxury of warm weather all year round. They often run indoors on hard, unforgiving surfaces. These hard surfaces do not absorb any shock or force. Consequently, the foot, ankle, and lower leg absorb the entire force. Always encourage your son or daughter to run on forgiving surfaces like grass or a running track whenever possible.

Another cause of shin splints is poor conditioning before the start of an athlete's sport season. Many spring sport athletes, for example, do not compete in winter sports activities, such as basketball. Some may come to track-and-field practice out of shape. They lack strength, flexibility, endurance, and agility. They immediately go full speed into sprinting and jumping, and their bodies cannot keep up. The result is often injury. Encourage your son or daughter to run before the track season begins. Running for one week before practice starts is not enough. Allow several weeks to a few months to condition the body.

Anatomical differences can also cause shin splints. Athletes who have excessively pronated feet, regardless of the reason, are at greater risk for shin splints. Extreme pronation causes stress to the muscles and tendons that provide support to the arch. Excessively tight calf muscles, for example, can cause shin splints.

Other factors include muscle imbalance, knee alignment, and foot structure. A physician, physical therapist, or certified athletic trainer can evaluate these conditions.

Shin splint treatments will vary from one person to the next. What works for one person may not work for another. Therefore, you may want to try several of the following treatments. Do not be discouraged if one approach does not work:

- Modify your child's training. Running fewer miles on more forgiving surfaces and allowing the body to rest may help alleviate shin splints. Allow athletes to increase their mileage by only 10 percent per week, especially at the beginning of the season. This allows the body to accommodate to the added stress.
- Change shoes when appropriate.
- Try ice. Ice massage seems to work very well, as does a cold whirlpool before and after practices or games. Refer to the Evaluation, Treatment, and Prevention chapter for different methods of icing.
- Consult a physician. Your doctor may rule out any anatomical causes for your son's shin splints. He or she may suggest an anti-inflammatory medication, and might also refer you to a physical therapist or athletic trainer for other recommendations.

Stress Fractures

Every time we walk or run, we stress our bones. Normally, bone responds to this stress by building more bone on top of itself through a complicated physiological process. This strengthens the bone and allows us to maintain our active lifestyle. But if we run too much and do not allow our bodies to complete this bone-building process, our bones can become weak. They may even break if we continue to stress them without treating the injury. The first diagnosed stress fractures were found among military trainees. The fractures were caused by a combination of improper footwear and repeated physical stress.

Here is a simple exercise to help you understand how a stress fracture happens. First, take a wire coat hanger from your closet. In the middle of the hanger base, bend the coat hanger a few times in the same place. After several seconds, touch the spot you were bending. It should feel warm, even hot. In our bodies, when we place stress on a bone, the body heats the affected area. The increase in heat is the body saying, "Help! I need more bone!" If you continue to bend the coat hanger, it breaks. In our bodies, if we do not allow our bones enough of a chance to rebuild, we risk stress fractures that can lead to complete fractures.

Stress fractures can happen anywhere, but most happen in the lower leg and are the result of overuse. Because of hormonal and anatomical differences (wider hips, larger Q-angle in the knee), women are more susceptible to stress fractures than men.

Stress fractures often have the same symptoms as shin splints, but there are some key differences:

- Rest relieves pain. This was obvious in our coat hanger experiment. When we stopped bending the coat hanger, the hot wire began to cool. Similarly, when we remove the stress on the bone, the pain goes away. Stress fracture patients experience pain *during* exercise, whereas shin splint pain comes on *after* activity.
- The pain is almost unbearable with stress fractures. Athletes with shin splints can often treat their injuries symptomatically—with ice, Advil, and so forth—and remain competitive. People with stress fractures cannot. They require rest. Touching the bone, even very lightly, will cause excruciating pain if your son or daughter has a stress fracture. Stress fracture patients can usually point to the area or areas that hurt the most. Shin splint patients, on the other hand, have more soft tissue pain than bone pain.

You will need to refer your child to a physician if you suspect a stress fracture. Most stress fractures do not show up on x-ray for many weeks. A bone scan is required to diagnose stress fractures. Just as we detected heat in our coat hanger experiment, a bone scan detects heat in our bones. Rest is the only treatment for stress fractures. If your daughter has a lower-leg stress fracture, she may be able to pursue other forms of conditioning, like swimming, to stay in shape.

Achilles Injuries

Achilles tendonitis is another common ailment among athletes. We have all heard of a particular problem or weak area called an "Achilles heel." This term refers to the ancient Greek warrior, Achilles, whose only area of vulnerability was said to be his heel. The Achilles tendon is the long, thick cord in the back of the heel. It connects the calf muscles to the heel bone and allows us to stand on our toes.

Runners, dancers, soccer players, and basketball players suffer a large proportion of injuries to the Achilles tendon area. Usually, these injuries occur because athletes wear ill-fitting shoes or they train improperly (they might run too far too soon and without adequate warm-up). In many cases, a person's physical structure can predispose him or her to injury. Excessively flat feet, for example, can cause Achilles problems.

Achilles injuries can range from a slight irritation to a complete tendon rupture. Most injuries occur just an inch or two above where the Achilles connects to the heel bone, although this injury can happen anywhere on the tendon.

Achilles tendonitis (where the Achilles tendon is inflamed, but not ruptured) is especially common in children. The injury usually starts out mild and gets progressively worse as the young athlete continues to play. This is when you need to ask athletes the "W" questions: "When did this start bothering you?" "What kind of pain is this?" "Where (specifically) does it hurt?" They will almost always say that it hurts on the tendon and that it has gradually become worse. The tendon is tender or painful when pressed or pinched. It may feel warmer than the other, uninjured Achilles tendon. This happens because the body heats the area in an effort to promote the healing process. This, too, is an indication of possible injury.

While it is possible to rupture the Achilles tendon, this injury is most common to athletes over thirty. It is usually not a problem with young athletes. When the tendon does rupture, athletes will often feel as if they have been shot in the heel. Many people even turn around to find the gunman! Because the tendon ruptures, most people find it nearly impossible to walk. Swelling, bruising, and discomfort in the calf muscles follow the initial severe pain.

If an Achilles tendon ruptures, refer the athlete to a physician immediately. Surgical treatment is often required to restore normal function to the lower leg. With or without surgery, the rehabilitation process is lengthy—three to six months.

If you suspect your child has Achilles tendonitis (where the tendon is inflamed, but not ruptured), there are simple treatments you can try at home. The injury requires relative rest from painful activities. We all know active people who view rest as failure, but avoiding pain-causing activities is good medicine.

Ice and elevation will reduce swelling and inflammation. Apply ice several times per day to reduce pain. Remember that a bag of frozen vegetables works great!

Gently stretch the Achilles tendon to help keep the joint mobile. In addition, using a heel lift (available at your local pharmacy) will elevate the heel and reduce stress to the tendon. Heel lifts work well for some people and not so well for others. They are an inexpensive, conservative treatment, however, so if they do not work for your son or daughter, you have not wasted too much money.

It is important to treat the cause as well as the symptoms of an Achilles injury. Consult with a physician, physical therapist, or athletic trainer in your area for an evaluation. These people can determine specific causes and make recommendations to prevent reinjury.

Compartment Syndrome

Earlier in this chapter, we discussed the compartments of the lower leg. These compartments hold the muscles, blood vessels, and nerves of the lower leg. When we injure any of the compartments, we risk injury to the other tissues as well.

When an athlete is kicked in the lower leg, bleeding occurs in the injured tissues. Usually, we do not even know the bleeding is happening. Almost always, the injury appears as a minor bruise. However, sometimes the bleeding occurs deep inside the compartment(s). Because these compartments are separated by tissue, the bleeding will often stay inside one compartment. This causes pressure inside the compartment to increase, blocking the vessels and putting pressure on the nerves inside the leg. This, in turn, creates more pressure inside of the compartment, creating a vicious cycle.

There are two types of compartment syndrome—acute and recurrent. Acute compartment syndrome requires immediate medical attention. The pressure inside the compartment can stop normal blood flow and normal nerve function to the rest of the lower leg.

Refer to the following list of red flags to determine if your son or daughter may be suffering from acute compartment syndrome:

- The area is very painful, and it feels hard to the touch. This will most likely occur in the front of the lower leg, but acute compartment syndrome can happen anywhere.
- Pointing the foot and toes down causes pain.
- The patient complains of numbness in the web space between the first and second toe. This indicates nerve involvement. If this is present, go immediately to the emergency room.
- Any numbness or decreased sensation to the foot, lower leg, or toes. This is another indication of possible nerve involvement and is equally serious.
- Pain and other symptoms that do not disappear when your child stops activity.

If any of these symptoms appear, contact your physician immediately. Early treatment is always best here.

Recurrent compartment syndrome is much more common than acute compartment syndrome. It is not caused by trauma, but by overuse (thus, it has a close resemblance to shin splints). While it may be painful, it is much less painful than acute compartment syndrome. The compartment does not have the same hardness, and the sensation in the legs and feet is normal. In addition, the pain and other symptoms disappear when your child stops activity. Because these symptoms resemble shin splints, you should consult with your physician about your concerns. In any case, a professional trained in sports medicine should evaluate any lower leg pain that lasts longer than several days.

Again, ice will help reduce pain and inflammation—get out that bag of frozen peas! Running on different surfaces (like grass), wearing different shoes, and stretching the muscles of the lower leg can help treat or prevent these injuries.

Ankle Injuries

An ankle sprain is an injury to one or more of the ligaments in the ankle. Some of these ligaments connect the tibia to the fibula, others connect the tibia and fibula to different bones in the foot. The ligaments on the inside of the ankle are stronger and injured less often than the ligaments on the outside of the ankle. We determine the severity of an ankle sprain by assessing the ligaments involved. Most ankle sprains occur on the outside of the ankle and happen when the foot is pointed, like when someone steps on an opponent's foot in basketball. Sports in which players cut back and forth or change directions often—like basketball, football, and soccer—are notorious for these injuries. Ankle injuries are also common in field sports, because the playing surface is often uneven.

Right Foot and Ankle (viewed from the right side)

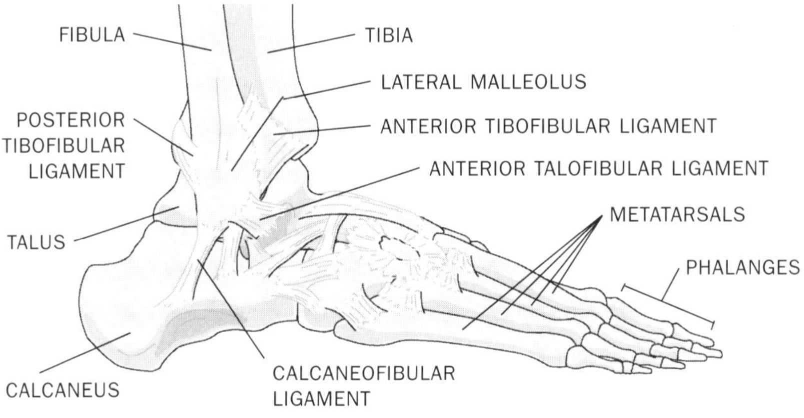

Athletes with sprained ankles often say they "rolled their ankle over." This injury is very common, especially in sports like basketball or football. Opponents jump for a ball, and one lands on the other's foot, causing the foot to turn inward. This damages the ligaments on the outside of the foot (which connect the fibula to the talus and the calcaneus).

Some athletes who sprain their ankle hear a "pop" or "crack." This sound does not necessarily indicate an ankle fracture (broken bone). Tearing ligament fibers can also cause the pop or crack.

Depending on their severity, ankle sprains can cause minimal amounts of pain, or they can be excruciating. Excruciating injuries may require surgery. Remember that ankle sprains are injuries to the ligaments, not the bones. An x-ray is the only way to rule out a fracture, but pressing on a ligament sprain should cause pain over the ligament, not the bone.

Because of the pain, athletes may be unable to bear weight, causing them to limp. This may not indicate the severity of the injury, however, especially in young and adolescent children. Often, these children have not yet experienced a true injury, and their fear may cause the limp associated with pain. Noting the limp is very good information for the person evaluating the injury, however.

With an ankle sprain, the ankle is weak because of the pain involved with the injury. Most ankle sprains do not cause nerve damage, but they may cause muscle injury. In this case, the athlete feels pain throughout the foot, not just over the ligament.

An ankle sprain causes some degree of swelling. While this may look grotesque to a concerned mother or father, the swelling is a normal response. Many injuries often look much worse than they are. For that reason, wait for a physician's evaluation before assuming the worst, especially if the swelling looks severe.

Minor sprains require only ten days to two weeks to heal, while sprains that are more significant require much longer. Ankle sprains that are properly treated get better much more quickly than those that receive little or no treatment. To treat an ankle sprain properly, monitor it carefully. Consult with your physician. He or she will rule out fractures, which are more significant than sprains, and assist you with an order for physical therapy.

Apply RICE immediately. Remember that RICE stands for Rest, Ice, Compression, and Elevation. Apply a cold pack as soon as possible for ten to fifteen minutes. A bag of frozen peas works very well. We tell our young patients that if they use the frozen peas for their injuries, Mom and Dad cannot make them eat them! An ACE bandage provides excellent compression. When applying the ACE bandage, wrap it from the bottom of the injury to the top. This prevents the swelling from moving into the foot and toes. Elevating the injury will also prevent the swelling from going into the rest of the foot.

Never apply heat to an acute ankle sprain (an ankle sprain that just happened). This will make the swelling much worse. Heat will open the blood vessels and allow a lot of unwanted fluid into the area. This excess fluid limits range of motion and increases the time required for the injury to get better. Heat is beneficial after the first seventy-two hours, when used with alternating cold-hot-cold-hot treatments. You will never go wrong with ice, however. This is true for most injuries in this book.

Crutches may be helpful for an athlete with a sprained ankle. People, especially children, assume the worst when they see crutches. Some view crutches as a sympathy tool, while others think only catastrophic injuries require crutches. In reality, crutches may enable your son or daughter to walk more effectively without causing excessive stress to the injury.

It is difficult to walk over uneven surfaces with a sprained ankle, because the ligaments that normally provide stability are damaged. Explain to your child or player that walking on surfaces like snow or grass may cause even more damage, and this can delay his or her recovery. Furthermore, walking from side to side is more difficult than walking forward.

Your athlete should start some type of rehabilitation program after an ankle sprain. The program should include stretching and strengthening exercises, as well as exercises to help increase his or her balance and awareness of surroundings. Standing on one foot, first with the eyes open, then with the eyes closed, is a good exercise for this. Ankle rehabilitation is quite easy, and most patients improve quickly. Technique and dedication are the keys. A physical therapist or certified athletic trainer can teach your son or daughter the proper exercise techniques, but you must encourage the child to stick to them. Exercises may not be fun, so dedication is essential.

Strengthening the muscles of the lower leg is important after a sprained ankle, because the damaged ligaments cannot work as effectively as they did before the injury. Strong muscles, however, can provide the necessary stability. Strengthening exercises should not cause pain. Stretching exercises are equally important. Some muscles and tendons in the lower leg, such as the Achilles tendon, will tighten to help stabilize the joint. These need to stretch out before exercise.

Taping or bracing the injured ankle is necessary to provide more stability following the initial injury. Many sporting goods stores and pharmacies carry ankle braces. We especially recommend the Swede-O ankle brace. It provides ankle stability, and users lace up the brace just like they would lace up a shoe. This makes the brace very efficient. Taping the ankle is also effective; however, the skill of the person applying the tape determines its effectiveness. A certified athletic trainer is the best person for this job.

It can be difficult to recognize the difference between an ankle sprain and an ankle fracture. In fact, an x-ray is often required to identify a fracture. The following are some very basic, though not foolproof, ways to differentiate between the two.

Athletes who fracture an ankle often sprain or damage the ligaments in the ankle as well. Both fractures and sprains cause muscle strength to reduce significantly.

With a fracture, swelling is usually localized, and patients feel a lot of pain on the bone. Ligament injuries, on the other hand, do not typically cause as much pain on the bone area.

Severe fractures can disrupt normal blood flow and nerve signals. When assessing an ankle injury, always determine the skin color in the area below the injury, and ask the injured athlete to wiggle his or her toes. If the foot is turning blue, or the player cannot move his or her toes, a fracture may have caused nerve or blood-supply damage. This requires a trip to the doctor or emergency room.

With ankle sprains, most experts agree that immobilizing the ankle causes more problems than it solves. Your physician may brace the injury for a period of time, but most people do not require a lower leg cast for an ankle sprain. Some fractures, however, require casting and immobilization.

Toe Injuries

Toe injuries can be very painful. If you have ever stubbed your toe so badly that the toenail falls off, you know what we are talking about. Toes injuries can affect the way we walk down the hall or up and down the stairs.

Injuries to the toes can involve ligaments, bones, tendons, and other tissues. It is possible, then, that injuries to these tissues will cause a lot of pain. The big toe (also called the great toe) plays an important role in how we walk and run. It also bears most of the weight. For this reason, injuries to the great toe cause more problems than injuries to other toes.

In this section, we will highlight several common injuries to the toes and offer basic treatment ideas.

Turf Toe

"Turf toe" is a common injury to the big toe. It is a ligament injury often caused by excessive toe extension (like when the toe points up) and other excessive movements. Fans of the National Football League often hear announcers discuss a player's turf toe injury. Many people assume that players have to compete on artificial turf to suffer this injury. This is not true. Although it is common for athletes who play on artificial turf to have this injury, it can happen to virtually any athlete involved in running sports.

Turf toe injuries are painful, although the degree of pain depends on the degree of the injury. Pain can range from the very mild to the very severe, limiting normal walking and other functions. Pushing off with the foot or toe causes the most pain. In fact, some people walk like a duck when they have this injury. Depending on the degree of injury, there may be some swelling around the joint where the toe joins the foot.

To treat turf toes injuries:

- Consult with your physician. A doctor will rule out any other injuries, like fractures to the joint. He or she may also recommend medication and other treatment ideas.
- Ice. Because this is a soft tissue injury, ice helps reduce the pain and swelling.

- Avoid strenuous activities that overwork the joint. Running five to ten miles with turf toe may not cause life-long problems, but it will aggravate the injury and delay the healing process.
- Purchase a turf toe strap. This adhesive-backed material limits excessive movement of the toe. It is cost effective, simple to use, and athletes usually do not require help putting them on. An orthotic is another option (see below). For more information on either of these products, contact a physician or certified athletic trainer.

Bunions

This is a common disorder of the toe. Bunions are easy to assess, because the great toe points toward the outside of the foot. Bunion patients have large bumps on the sides of their feet, near the big toe joint. With this injury, there is usually a callus on the skin near the joint, and the bursa sac inside the joint is thick. Bunions affect women more then men because women typically wear tight-fitting shoes, like high heels and other dress shoes. Improper footwear does not cause all bunions, however. Many people "inherit" bunions through genetics.

Bunions can be very painful. If we drive a car when its tires are out of alignment, the tires wear quickly, compromising the safety of the passengers. The same is true with bunions. The joint does not work efficiently. This inefficiency causes pain and can create difficulty with other daily activities.

There are, however, many ways to treat these injuries:

- Wear wide shoes. Giving the foot and toe enough room will relieve the stress to the joint and allow the patient greater mobility. Athletic shoes are a good choice for bunion patients, because they give the feet plenty of room.
- RICE painful joints. This is an efficient, inexpensive way to reduce pain.
- Contact your physician. A doctor may recommend orthotics to reduce the pain. Orthotics vary in length and construction.

Physical therapists, podiatrists, and orthotist will typically make orthotics to fit the specific needs of your athlete. Occasionally, doctors may recommend surgical treatment.

Foot Injuries

Earlier, we discussed the bones and muscles in the foot. Ligaments hold the bones together, and tendons attach the muscles to the bones. Because the anatomy is so complex, injuries are common. We will discuss a few of these here.

Neuroma

Neuroma is a nerve injury in which the metatarsals pinch the nerves of the foot. The nerves thicken as a result of the pinching. Because tight-fitting shoes seem to cause this, women are predisposed to these injuries. Touching the area between the bones in the ball of the foot causes pain, and you may feel a tender knot in that area. Most often, neuroma patients will be unable to put weight on their feet if they have tight-fitting shoes. Therefore, to prevent these injuries, encourage your athletes to wear shoes that do not compress the foot.

Treatment of neuroma varies. Many patients find relief from an orthotic or arch support. These will relieve pressure on the pinched nerves. Some physicians recommend physical therapy and anti-inflammatory medication to reduce inflammation and pain. Anti-inflammatory medications do not correct the problems that cause the pinching, however, so it is best to solve the underlying problems instead of masking them. Your physician may recommend surgery to remove the neuroma. If he or she recommends this, be certain to ask if more conservative efforts would help first.

Metatarsal Fracture

The metatarsal bones (the small bones between the ball of the foot and the phalanges) can break just like any other bones. Athletes involved in running, soccer, football, basketball, and tennis are particularly susceptible to these injuries. Pain is usually located directly on the bone, and activity usually increases the pain.

Consider arch supports or a custom-fitted orthotic to relieve stress to the bones. If all else fails, rest is the ideal treatment.

Sesamoiditis

Sesamoid bones are the little bones in the ball of the foot (see page 98). Sesamoiditis causes pain at the ball of the foot, just below the big toe. Pressing on the joint causes moderate to severe pain. Bearing weight is typically difficult, and pushing off (when running or cutting) is extremely difficult. Pulling the toe up (toward the head) may cause pain, because this motion compresses the bone.

Treatment varies with sesamoiditis. Ice relieves pain, and orthotics may relieve pressure to the area. For example, Craig was a high-profile basketball player who had sesamoiditis. A physical therapist made custom-fitted orthotics for him, and his pain was gone within ten days. For him, this was all the treatment he needed. Anti-inflammatory medication may also reduce pain and inflammation, particularly when used in conjunction with physical therapy. Contact your doctor regarding all medication questions.

Navicular Fractures and Accessory Naviculars

The navicular (scaphoid) bone, which is located on the inside of the foot, is the point of attachment for the muscles on the inside of the foot (see page 98). Navicular fractures require a cast, and some require surgery. These injuries take a long time to heal.

Most people have one navicular in each foot. Some people, however, have two naviculars in one or both feet. Less than 15 percent of the population suffers from this condition. Patients with an accessory navicular often experience little—if any—pain, but jumping and cutting sports may cause discomfort. In some cases, the discomfort can cause a limp. Because the accessory bone rubs against the inside of the shoe, a callus can form over the bone. The bump may turn red because of the rubbing.

Rest and ice will reduce pain, soreness, and inflammation to the tendons that insert on the accessory bone. Athletes should also choose footwear that doesn't put a lot of pressure on the area. Arch supports provide relief for some people. Lifting the arch reduces stress on the tendons and ligaments surrounding the bone. In theory, this will reduce pain. For many people, this provides great relief. For others, the relief is only minimal. If all else fails, surgical removal of the accessory bone will correct the problem.

Flat Feet

Flat feet, also known as excessive pronation, can cause several problems, although not all flat-footed people will experience them. Clearly, flat feet are not optimal. Because the arches have fallen, more stress is placed upon the ligaments and tendons in the foot. This, in turn, creates an unstable, flexible foot. All of this makes the foot more prone to injury.

Orthotics, arch supports, strengthening exercises, and wearing proper shoes can profoundly influence a person's level of comfort. One exercise we give patients is called the "towel crunch." To do this exercise, simply place a towel on the floor and curl it with your toes. Pulling the towel toward you with each crunch strengthens the muscles in the foot and arch. We also instruct people to purchase shoes that control the motion at the arch. Many running shoes call this "motion control." Unfortunately, these shoes are seldom in the $9.99 clearance bin at your local Target or Wal-Mart. They cost more money, but they provide more relief.

It is impossible to say that flat feet are of no concern. However, many athletes (even professional athletes) compete with flat feet everyday. Your child can do the same.

High Arches

High arches, also known as excessive supination, are the opposite of flat feet. Patients with high arches have very rigid feet that do not absorb shock very well. If a car has poor shocks, the passengers feel every bump in the road. Similarly, if the feet absorb shock poorly, the force is transferred to the rest of the leg, and this can cause injury. Injuries such as tendonitis and stress fractures often result from feet that do not absorb force or shock properly.

This is a highly-manageable condition. The key is to treat the injury symptomatically. In other words, treat the injury for its symptoms (pain, swelling, etc.). Choose shoes specifically designed to absorb shock. Your athlete may also require a shock-absorbing orthotic or insert for his or her shoes.

Flat feet and feet with high arches are often genetic conditions. Other causes include previous injury and, for flat feet, obesity.

Heel Injuries

Calcaneal Apophysitis

Adolescent athletes, especially those in running and jumping sports, sometimes suffer from a condition called calcaneal apophysitis. The pain generally starts as a dull ache in the back of the heel and increases with activities involving the calf muscles (like lifting the heel off the ground). The area around the Achilles tendon may swell. Fortunately, this condition does not usually affect daily activities.

This injury normally happens near the area of the bone where growing occurs. Because of this, the condition improves when the athlete stops growing.

Calcaneal apophysitis requires evaluation by a physician. Ice reduces inflammation and relieves pain. Eliminating the offensive activity also reduces pain. Furthermore, gentle, pain-free stretching of the Achilles tendon and calf muscles can decrease the stress to the area. The operative words here are "gentle" and "pain-free."

Bruises and Heel Spurs

A heel spur is a growth of bone on the heel. A heel bruise is a bruise to the fat pad of the heel. Both cause considerable pain. Because their symptoms look like other heel injuries (plantar fasciitis, for example), you will want to have a physician take an x-ray. Patients with heel spurs or heel bruises experience pain when they walk on their heels.

Plantar Fasciitis

The plantar fascia is the soft tissue that provides support to the arch and runs along the bottom of the foot from the heel to the toes. Plantar fasciitis has become a common injury in the 1990s, and you may even know someone with this injury. Excessively high arches or flat feet seem to contribute to this injury.

If your son often complains about foot pain between his arch and heel bone, think about the following. Plantar fasciitis pain usually begins in the heel after excessive walking or running. People often complain that the first few steps (like after getting out of bed in the morning) cause tremendous pain. In fact, one patient almost did not make it to the bathroom in the middle of the night because his foot hurt too much to walk. (Fortunately, he made it!) It is foolish to allow a young athlete to play when symptoms reach this extreme.

Use RICE to treat this injury, and consult with a physical therapist or certified athletic trainer regarding the proper footwear. The correct shoe can prevent injury, but the "wrong" shoe can actually cause injury. Some athletes, though not all, find relief simply by changing their shoes.

Anti-inflammatory medication will reduce the inflammation and help control the pain. Physical therapy may also help. Ask a doctor if this would benefit your child or player. A physical therapist or athletic trainer can work with your son to improve range of motion in his foot, which will reduce the stress to the plantar fascia. He or she may also recommend strengthening exercises to prevent reinjury, and/or a splint to wear at night to help stretch the plantar fascia while your son sleeps.

Finding the Right Shoes

Because feet vary so much between individuals, a shoe for one person may not work well for another. For your information, we have identified several components of the shoe to help you determine whether or not a particular shoe is appropriate for your child.

The midsole is probably the most crucial part of the shoe. Individuals with high arches require a flexible midsole. This type of shoe absorbs shock better, and people with high arches need that added shock absorption. In contrast, people with flat feet require a more rigid midsole because they lack stability in their arches. A rigid midsole provides this stability.

The outersole makes contact with the ground. Wear patterns on the outersole indicate how the foot strikes the ground. For example, excessive wear on the outside of the shoe may indicate high, rigid arches. In this case, try a shoe with a flexible midsole. A person with flat feet may have wear on the inside of the shoe. In this case, try a shoe with a rigid, more supportive midsole.

The toe box is where the toes and the ball of the foot rest. The size of the toe box varies from shoe to shoe. Patients with bunions and neuromas require a wide toe box. High heels, however, have a very narrow toe box.

Depending on the type of shoe, the heel can either stabilize the foot or provide shock absorption. If your athlete has high arches, go for the shock absorption. Athletes with flat feet, on the other hand will want stability.

Contact a physical therapist or athletic trainer in your area if you have any questions regarding these components. They can refer you to someone who is knowledgeable about shoes and can sell you a shoe that meets your needs.

Conclusion

Injuries to the foot, ankle, and lower leg are quite common among younger (and older) athletes. Most injuries result from overuse or poor training techniques, like running too far without adequate preparation. However, certain shoes can cause injuries. Runners should change shoes at least every year to year-and-a-half, or four hundred to five hundred miles, whichever comes first.

Ice and rest will frequently resolve the symptoms. Athletes can usually compete effectively if they ice their injuries after practices and games. However, ice does not address the cause of an injury. Try some of the ideas we discuss in this chapter (like stretching well and changing shoes or running surfaces). You may also wish to contact a physical therapist or an athletic trainer in your area for more advice. As always, your physician can refer you to a medical specialist who will address your concerns and problems.

Frequently Asked Questions

Q: *My daughter just got out of a cast. She broke her ankle. What should she concentrate on now?*

A: She should concentrate on range of motion. Regaining lost range of motion is important and can be a difficult process. In addition, encourage your daughter to remain as active as possible. Riding an exercise bike, doing upper-body stretching and strengthening exercises (when appropriate) and maintaining a positive outlook is important when coming out of a cast.

One exercise we like is the alphabet exercise. To do this, your daughter should lay on her back with her foot and ankle elevated with a pillow or two. Then, ask her to write the alphabet in the air, pretending that her foot is a pen. Once she regains her range of motion, she can begin gentle strengthening exercises. The joint will be stiff. Isometric strengthening—like pushing against a wall or an immovable object—is safe and effective. Some other strengthening exercises require the use of flexible tubing. The tubing is color-coded based on level of resistance, so you should consult with your physician, physical therapist, or athletic trainer regarding its use. If either of these recovery phases is too difficult, your physician may recommend therapy so that your daughter receives the best possible care.

Q: *How long do sprained ankles take to heal?*

A: It varies. Some take less than one week, others can take several weeks. The best way to minimize the effects of an ankle sprain is to treat the injury when it happens. Waiting several days can delay recovery time drastically. Remember the RICE principle and make sure you contact an athletic trainer or physical therapist for exercises.

Q: *My daughter is a runner, and she has a fibular stress fracture. She thinks that she can "tough it out." Am I insane, or is this impossible?*

A: Your physician has probably ordered her in a walking cast for up to six weeks, perhaps longer. This is good medicine. Do not let her "tough it out." Explain to her that stress fractures lead to complete fractures. Kids think they're invincible, but you have the executive power to limit her activity.

Q: *Are shin splints inevitable? My son can't seem to get rid of them.*

A: No. Contact your physician. He or she can order anti-inflammatory medication and prescribe physical therapy and/or orthotics. Also, try simple things, like changing shoes as well as the surface on which your son runs. Shin splints can be extremely painful, but there are effective treatment options available.

Q: *My son's ankle hurts when he plays soccer. Should he get a brace for it?*

A: Yes. He should have a brace or find an athletic trainer to tape his ankle. The pain is most likely from weak lower leg muscles that cannot stabilize his ankle joint. If your son strengthens those lower leg muscles, this should take away the problem. We recommend Swede-O ankle braces for our patients. A sporting goods store should carry these braces. If not, contact a physical therapy clinic in your area. They may order one for you.

Contributing Author: Kecia Sell, MS, PT, ATC

Kecia is a certified athletic trainer and physical therapist with Fairview Rehabilitation Services, where she also serves as Manager of Clinical Operations. Kecia teaches the principles of rehabilitation (especially regarding foot, ankle, and lower leg injuries) to medical professionals throughout the country. Kecia and her husband, Jim, have one son, Jordan, age two.

Contributing Author: Jill McCartney, PT

Jill is a physical therapist with the Institute for Athletic Medicine, St. Anthony Clinic, where she specializes in treating patients with foot and ankle disorders. Jill also makes orthotics for IAM patients. She is also a therapist in the Running Program. Jill and her husband, Thomas, have one child, Abbey.

Contributing Author: Scott Kulstad, MEd, ATC/R

With Appreciation: Mary Hawley, PT, and Susie Oster, PT

Chapter

7

The Knee

At virtually every public speaking or community education event that we participate in, parents, athletes, and coaches ask us about knee injuries. High profile professional athletes, such as Robert Smith (Minnesota Vikings), Ki Jana Carter (Cincinnati Bengals), and Danny Manning (Phoenix Suns) have all suffered knee injuries. Media attention to their injuries has created a spotlight on all knee injuries.

In the minds of many young athletes and their parents, even minor knee injuries seem like serious business. A young soccer player and her mother started crying even before I had evaluated her knee; they were certain that all knee injuries require surgery. In fact, the mother asked if I would recommend a good surgeon to perform "the procedure." In the end, the soccer player had a minor inflammation that went away within two or three days. Knee injuries are common in sports like football, soccer, skiing, gymnastics, and basketball.

Because of their structure, women seem to be more vulnerable to chronic knee injuries than men. As your daughter matures, her hips widen in preparation for possible childbirth. This can change the way her muscles act on her knees, causing added stress to the joints. Explain to your daughter that her hips widen because of the maturation process, and that she should not expect to slow or stop this process.

However, she can take the following steps to reduce her chances of injury:

- Strengthen the quadriceps (the muscles in the front of the thigh) and hamstrings (the muscles in the back). Striking a balance between these two muscle groups is important, so you may want to contact an athletic trainer in your area for specific suggestions on how to achieve this.
- Wear appropriate footwear for competition. This is good advice for both men and women. Many female athletes have had success with footwear designed especially for women.
- Maintain adequate conditioning levels throughout the season. People are at higher risk for injury when fatigue sets in.

Anatomy

Four bones make up the knee joint: the femur (the thighbone), the tibia (the shinbone), the fibula (the smaller bone on the outside of the lower leg), and the patella (the kneecap). The femur is very large, and portions of this bone create the bulge on the outside of the knee. The tibia creates the plateau surface on which the femur glides. For that reason, we consider the knee a "hinge joint." Its primary movements are extending (straightening) and flexing (bending) the leg.

The patella is a "floating" bone and acts like a pulley mechanism to control knee motion. The patella glides in a groove within the thighbone, forming another joint in the knee—called the patellofemoral joint—which is created by the patella and the femur. Injuries to this joint are very common, and we will discuss them in depth later.

Four major ligaments connect all the bones but the patella. Two collateral ligaments are located on the sides of the knee: the lateral collateral ligament (LCL) is on the outside of the knee, and the medial collateral ligament (MCL) is on the inside of the knee. Two other ligaments cross inside the knee joint; they are called cruciate ligaments. The most famous ligament in the knee is the anterior cruciate ligament (ACL). People fear injury to this ligament because surgical reconstruction is the most common treatment. The posterior cruciate ligament (PCL) is also inside the knee. It crosses behind the ACL.

Right Knee, Bending (viewed from the front)

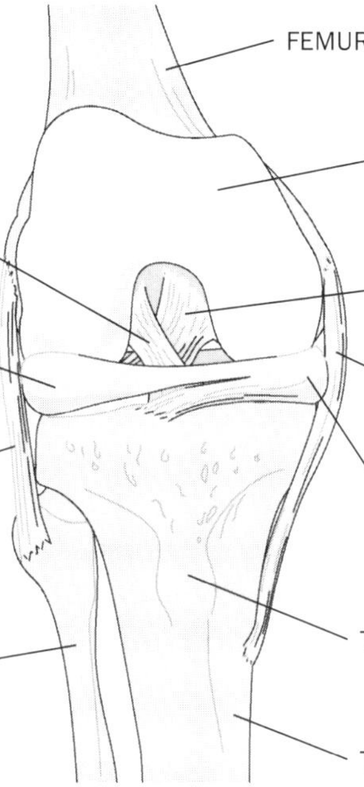

Many different muscles act on the knee. The quadriceps muscles in the front of the thigh straighten the knee, and the hamstring muscles in the back of the thigh bend the knee. We discuss these muscles in detail in the Pelvis, Hip, and Thigh chapter. However, keep in mind that the inside quadriceps muscle—called the VMO—is particularly important. The VMO helps extend (straighten) the knee and move the kneecap properly in its place.

Other structures play important roles within the knee as well. Inside the knee rests cartilage (meniscus) that supports and cushions the joint when we walk, run, and play. Injuries to the meniscus can influence the health of the knee joint throughout life. Surrounding the knee is a joint capsule that provides stability and lubrication. A different cartilage, called hyaline cartilage, lines the surface of the joints. This cartilage is different from the meniscus.

Ligament Injuries

The anterior cruciate ligament, commonly known as the ACL, is the primary stabilizer of the knee. Because this ligament is so important to the knee, injuries to the ACL often require surgical treatment.

ACL tears result from twisting or hyperextending the knee (when the knee is forcibly straightened too much). These injuries result from traumatic or forceful movements, not from repetitive activities. Athletes with ACL tears often say that their foot remained fixed to the ground while their knee twisted or hyperextended. This seems especially true among athletes who play on artificial turf, which tends to be more rigid than a natural surface.

Only medical professionals can determine the integrity of an ACL after a knee injury, and even they sometimes depend on diagnostic tests, like an MRI, to know for sure. However, you should keep the following in mind. Most ACL injuries swell rapidly and extensively. Within a few minutes to an hour, the knee is very swollen. Furthermore, most ACL injuries hurt a lot. Athletes complain of sharp, burning pain inside the joint. Many patients say they heard or felt a "pop" or "snap" when the injury occurred. This sound does not always indicate a ligament tear, but it is great information for the physician or athletic trainer who is evaluating the injured knee. When Dave tore his ACL, he heard five loud "pops," and his friends heard them as well.

Because the ACL provides stability to the joint, tearing the ligament makes the knee feel wobbly, loose, or prone to "give way." In fact, patients often say that when the injury happened, they felt their knee give way.

Medial collateral ligament (MCL) injuries happen when an athlete is hit on the outside of the knee, causing stress to the inside of the knee. This happens a lot in football, like when an opponent falls on a lineman's knee, or when a running back is tackled at the knee. It can also happen in sports like soccer and basketball when players twist their knees. As with an ACL injury, the joint feels unstable. There is pain on the inside portion of the knee, and athletes can usually point to the location of the pain.

Robert, a high-school football player, injured his MCL when another player fell on the outside of his knee. He had pain and some swelling, and his range of motion was limited. He could walk, but with a slight limp. He did not play football for five days. During that time, Robert strengthened his quadriceps muscles and followed the RICE principle. At the end of five days, he felt much better and was able to resume non-contact drills. He resumed full contact two days after that. Robert was lucky—his injury was a minor one.

Even when athletes severely injure their medial ligaments, they may not require surgery. Most players with severe injuries use knee braces and undergo physical therapy to strengthen the muscles of the quadriceps and hamstrings. Strong muscles provide the stability that injured ligaments cannot.

Lateral collateral ligament (LCL) injuries occur when an athlete is hit on the inside of the knee, causing stress to the outside of the knee. (This is the opposite of an MCL injury.) Athletes complain of pain and feel that their knee is unstable or loose. Many have mild to moderate swelling as well. Depending on the severity of the injury, bracing the knee allows athletes to resume competition. As with MCL injuries, physical therapy is a great treatment option. Ask your physician to recommend a good physical therapist or athletic trainer. He or she can monitor your child's progress and provide exercises to strengthen the knee.

Posterior cruciate ligament (PCL) injuries occur less frequently than other ligament injuries. The PCL is located behind the ACL. It is inside the knee joint. This ligament is often injured in car accidents when the bent knee hits the dashboard, but athletes will occasionally injure it while playing sports. In professional wrestling, for example, wrestlers jump off the "third rope" and land on their opponent with a bent knee. This may injure the PCL.

If your child injures his or her PCL, ask your doctor about treatment options, which should include physical therapy and possibly a brace for support. The RICE principle is a good idea as well.

Let's say you are watching your daughter's soccer game (perhaps you are even the coach), and she twists her knee. She lays on the field in obvious pain. Your job as a parent or coach is to properly manage the injury. The way you handle the injury can be either very comforting or very stressful to the athlete. First, calm the athlete. Instruct her to slowly breathe in through her nose and out through her mouth. Parents or coaches can help the athlete do this by breathing with her.

Stabilize the knee. When removing the athlete from the playing field, pay close attention to the injury. Avoid quick, jostling movements. Remember that removing the athlete from the field is not a race. Long-time Minnesota Vikings athletic trainer Fred Zamberletti says, "You don't need to break any land speed records getting the kid off." If you can stabilize the knee and get off the field slowly, the athlete will experience much less discomfort. In addition, you give his or her teammates a chance to rest.

After the incident, consult your physician. Knee injuries often require a physician's attention. In most cases, ligament injuries do not require a visit to the hospital or emergency room. Unless the athlete has uncontrollable pain, displays signs of shock, or appears to have extensive injury (tingling in his or her feet, intense bone pain, etc.), parents can contact the doctor's office the next day.

RICE—Rest, Ice, Compression, and Elevation—is an important part of treatment. The athlete obviously needs rest, and ice will help reduce swelling and control pain. An ACE bandage will also help control the swelling. Keep in mind, however, that because the knee swells rapidly, pressure inside the knee increases. If you wrap the ACE too tightly, the athlete may experience a throbbing pain because you have limited the body's ability to accommodate the pressure. Elevating the knee will reduce the swelling and discoloration that could move into the rest of the lower leg. We can thank gravity for that.

Meniscus Injuries

Inside the knee joint, there are two wedge-shaped pieces of cartilage called menisci (plural for meniscus). The meniscus is important because it provides stability and cushioning to the joint. Its surface allows the joint to bend smoothly. It also provides shock absorption, preventing the thighbone from crushing the shinbone when we walk and run. The medial meniscus, which is C-shaped, is secured to the knee joint. Because it lacks mobility, athletes often injure the cartilage. The meniscus on the outside of the knee has more mobility and is injured less often. Injuries to the meniscus occur when the foot is firmly planted on the ground and the bent knee twists. In all cases, injuries to this cartilage cause pain, swelling, locking, and clicking inside the knee. The joint also loses much of its range of motion. Unlike ligament injuries, meniscus injuries may not swell until twelve to twenty-four hours after the trauma.

Treatment of meniscus injuries usually includes surgery. The procedure is very common today, and patients are much better within a few weeks to a month or two following surgery. Erin was a sixteen-year-old basketball player who injured her medial meniscus. She had surgery on a Friday and resumed basketball practice three weeks later.

In this surgery, called an arthroscopy, surgeons use very tiny instruments (not much bigger than drinking straws) to remove the damaged pieces. Only a very small section of each meniscus has a blood supply, so its ability to heal itself is inefficient at best. This is why surgeons must remove damaged pieces.

If you suspect a meniscus injury, contact your physician as soon as possible. Early treatment allows athletes to resume their active lifestyle much sooner.

Kneecap Injuries

Injuries to the kneecap are either long-term (chronic) overuse injuries or sudden, acute injuries. An example of an acute injury would be falling on the kneecap while diving for a volleyball. A chronic injury, on the other hand, would start out very minor and gradually get worse over time. Most of the injuries young people have are chronic injuries.

Most, if not all, kneecap injuries cause pain and discomfort in the front of the knee. Your son may say that he has pain walking up and down stairs. He may also say that he cannot sit for long periods without knee pain, or that he cannot play sports without pain. Sports like running, soccer, basketball, and tennis are notorious for these injuries.

Structural problems in the knee cause most chronic pain. Tight or weak muscles can cause the kneecap to move incorrectly in its groove. Over time, this can cause degeneration of the hyaline cartilage, which lines the surface of the kneecap. (This cartilage is different from the meniscus, which is inside the knee joint.) Again, this is much like driving with your car out of alignment. Over time, the tires wear unevenly, and you have to fix the problem before the tires explode.

To understand the difference between ligament pain and patellar (kneecap) pain, think of the following. Kneecap pain occurs in the front of the knee. Ligament and meniscus injuries, on the other hand, cause pain on the joint line (where the thighbone meets the shinbone).

Kneecap pain does not usually cause significant swelling. If the patella feels watery and appears swollen (like a water balloon), your son may have injured the bursa sac that sits in the front of the knee. However, most patellofemoral joint injuries do not appear significantly swollen, whereas ligament and meniscus injuries typically cause swelling that is much more noticeable.

Unlike ligament injuries, kneecap injuries leave the joint feeling stable. The pain and discomfort usually subside with rest. Kneecap pain is more chronic than ligament pain. (Remember, ligament injuries are generally acute, occurring because of excessive force placed on the joint.) Not all pain that looks like kneecap pain should be dismissed as insignificant, however. There may be other, more serious reasons for your child's knee pain. All pain, especially pain that doesn't go away, should be addressed by a qualified medical professional.

Dislocated Kneecap

Another possible way to injure the knee is to dislocate the kneecap. In this type of injury, the kneecap slides out of its groove.

The injury is extremely painful and looks disgusting to the untrained eye. In fact, caring for a dislocated patella can be tricky, because the athlete is often more scared than anything else. In most patellar dislocations, the kneecap sits on the outside of the knee until a medical professional "puts it back in."

If this injury happens, your first objective is to evaluate the athlete and treat for shock (refer to the Emergency Procedures chapter). Assuming the athlete does not show signs of shock, you must calm the athlete. Immobilize the knee and seek medical attention immediately. If the athlete has extreme pain or has no way of riding comfortably to the emergency room, contact 911. Emergency response professionals can provide a much more comfortable ride, as well as medication to relieve the pain.

Fractures

Kneecap fractures sometimes occur in athletes who are hit directly on the knee, when they are tackled in football or hit with a slap shot in hockey, for example. In these sports, however, athletes wear protective kneepads, so kneecap fractures are uncommon. If you suspect a fractured kneecap, refer your child to an emergency facility immediately.

Other fractures to the knee are more common, particularly among athletes in heavy-contact sports. One specific fracture is called a tibial plateau fracture. This involves a traumatic break to the top surface of the tibia (shinbone). This injury requires immediate medical care. Follow the necessary steps (as discussed in the Emergency Procedures chapter) to transport the athlete to an emergency facility.

Jumper's Knee

Jumper's knee, or patellar tendonitis, is an inflammation of the patellar tendon, which is an extension of the quadriceps muscles. With your knee bent slightly, you can feel the patellar tendon, which is a chord-like tissue just below the kneecap. This tendon can become inflamed with repetitive jumping and landing activities, such as basketball or high jumping, and quick start-and-stop activities, like tennis.

The most common symptom of Jumper's Knee is pain along the tendon. The tendon may also appear slightly swollen, especially when compared with the uninjured leg. The best initial treatment you can give your son or daughter is RICE. Contact your physician for other recommendations.

Osgood-Schlatter's Disease

Osgood-Schlatter's Disease is very common among young people. Many experts believe that when children grow too quickly, the patellar tendon cannot keep up with the growth of the bone. Because of this, the tendon may pull away from the bone. When it pulls itself away from the bone, a portion of the bone comes with it. (This is called an avulsion fracture.) For that reason, most Osgood-Schlatter's patients have an obvious bump just below their patellar tendon.

This injury can cause mild to severe pain. Sports like basketball, high jump, and running can irritate this condition. In addition, your child may have difficulty walking up and down stairs and doing squats in the weight room. Contact your physician if you suspect your child has this condition. Most likely, he or she will recommend rest from the pain-causing activity and ice to control pain and inflammation. Anti-inflammatory medication may also relieve the pain and discomfort.

Baker's Cyst

A Baker's cyst (or popliteal cyst) is an inflammation of the bursa sac in the back of the knee. Most of these cysts are insignificant and can occur at any age for any reason. The cyst is usually not tender and does not limit function. The RICE principle works very well here. As grotesque as it may appear, it is a very mild injury that looks much worse than it really is.

ITB Syndrome

The iliotibial band is a lengthy tissue that starts near the hip and crosses the outside portion of the knee. Iliotibial band syndrome (ITB syndrome) is an inflammation of the part of the iliotibial band that crosses the knee. This injury is most common in runners.

Minor things can cause ITB syndrome, such as always running on the same side of the road. If your athlete runs on the same side of the road every day, the crown in the road will cause one leg to run at a different height than the other. Another possible cause is improper footwear. If your son has not changed shoes in over five hundred miles, consider buying him a new pair. (One woman had ITB syndrome for three months before she changed her shoes. Her problems were gone within a few weeks.) Muscle imbalances and excessively tight muscles can also cause ITB syndrome, so improving one's strength and flexibility can make a huge difference.

Conclusion

Knee pain can have several causes, including improper footwear, poor running surfaces, overuse, and acute injury. Furthermore, one injury can damage several different tissues. For example, in just one play during a soccer game, an athlete can twist her knee, tearing two ligaments and her meniscus. This is considered an acute injury. Most young athletes, however, suffer chronic pain as a result of an injury that occurs or worsens over a long period or time. Your decisions as a parent or coach will ultimately depend on the nature of the injury.

Chronic, long-term injuries do not require an urgent care or emergency room visit. Most are related to the kneecap joint. Chronic injuries will generally get better with only a few modifications to the person's daily routine. RICE and flexibility exercises will help. Contact your doctor for other suggestions, or consult with a physical therapist or athletic trainer to analyze possible causes for the injury (muscle imbalances, footwear, body structure, etc.).

Acute injuries happen because of a sudden twist or fall, as a result of being tackled, for example. Ligaments and menisci—the wedge-shaped cartilage inside the joint—are often injured in these scenarios. Unlike chronic injuries, acute injuries (such as ligament injuries) swell rapidly and significantly. Meniscus tears also swell, but they may take longer—sometimes up to twenty-four hours. In addition, meniscus tears cause clicking and popping, and may cause the knee to lock. Refer severe knee injuries to your family doctor or an orthopedic specialist for evaluation. Your doctor may elect to treat the injury with rest, physical therapy, or surgery.

In almost all cases, knee injuries are "fixable," and if your son or daughter wants to continue athletic participation, ask your physician for a referral to a physical therapist or athletic trainer. They are uniquely qualified to treat and manage knee injuries.

Frequently Asked Questions

Q: *My daughter's knees crack when she sits down. Should I be worried?*

A: No. Typically, we only tell people to worry about "little joint mice" when the cracking causes pain. If it does hurt, contact your doctor. The location of the crack and the type of pain it causes is particularly important. Creaking in the front of the knee is most likely related to the patellofemoral joint, while deep cracking may indicate meniscus damage.

Q: *My son can move his kneecap nearly an inch to the left or right. Is this normal?*

A: Yes. The patella has a tracking system that allows it to move from side to side. Some people can't move their patella as much as your son can move his, but this is normal, too.

Be aware that your son may have problems with his kneecap joint if he gets into highly competitive sports, such as basketball or track and field. If it doesn't hurt or cause problems, don't worry about fixing what isn't broken.

Q: *My daughter is in track, and she often has pain on the back of her knees after a run. What does this mean?*

A: It could indicate several things. One is that her hamstring muscles are tight and sore. These muscles attach in the back of the knee and are responsible for bending the knee—something we do a lot of when we run. There are smaller muscles in the back of the knee that could also be inflamed. Unless your daughter twisted her knee, it is unlikely that she has any serious injuries. Tell her to use RICE and to stretch her hamstrings. If the pain doesn't improve within a few days, make an appointment with your physician.

Contributing Author: Pam Bloedel, MPT

Pam is a physical therapist with the Institute for Athletic Medicine, Braemar Clinic. She specializes in treating a variety of sports-related injuries. She provides physical therapy to members of the Minnesota Timberwolves and Minnesota Twins. Pam and her husband, Shynne, recently had their first child, Keegan.

Contributing Author: Lee Bergstrom, PT, ATC/R

Lee is a certified athletic trainer and physical therapist with the Institute for Athletic Medicine, West Health Clinic, where she is also a supervisor. As a therapist in and coordinator of IAM's Running Program, Lee specializes in sports physical therapy. She holds a special interest in knee injuries because she is one of the statistics regarding serious knee injuries. Lee and her husband, Scott, have two children, Anna-Britt and David.

Chapter

8

The Pelvis, Hip, and Thigh

Many sports—perhaps all sports—involve the hips. Running, swimming, and even cycling sports rely on the hips. Because these sports require power and coordination, the hips must generate power in a very precise way. The pelvis, then, is also important, because the hip and thigh connect to the pelvis. If your son wants to punt a football, his foot must meet the ball with a lot of force and precise timing. If one of these components fails, his punt will not go far, or it may be blocked by an opponent. If a swimmer has weak hip muscles, she will be unable to propel herself through the water with speed. Her ability to succeed in and enjoy swimming, then, is based on the strength of her hips and thighs. In addition, her pelvis must be aligned correctly. Any deviation can result in injury or decreased level of performance.

Anatomy

The pelvis is a bony structure that connects the spine to the lower extremities. In fact, it is really three bones—the ilium, the ischium, and the pubis—fused into one. The pelvis serves as an attachment site for many muscles. It has many different parts, all playing an important role in hip motion and alignment of the back.

The ilium has several parts. The iliac crest, for example, forms the "ledge" of the pelvis. The anterior superior iliac spine (ASIS) is the prominent knob along the front of the iliac crest. People can see this when they stand in front of a mirror. Muscles and tendons insert on these portions. Because these muscles and tendons are so prominent, athletes in contact sports are at risk of injuring these structures. You may have heard of an injury called a "hip pointer." This is a bruise to the ASIS.

The ischium makes up the portion of the pelvis near the buttocks. The ischial tuberosity is very important. (A tuberosity is a portion of a bone that sticks out or serves as an attachment point for muscles and tendons.) Some people call the ischial tuberosity the "butt bone." The hamstring muscles (in the back of the thigh) insert here. People who sit too much sometimes get bursitis in this area. Bursitis is an inflammation of the ischial bursa sac. Pain, limited joint motion, and possible swelling characterize acute bursitis. RICE and anti-inflammatory medication are good treatments for this.

Just below the abdomen, the pubic bones (on each side of the body) form a junction called the pubic symphysis. Although this portion is generally immovable, it does move during childbirth. Direct contact (like being tackled in football) can cause injury to this area.

Where the three bones—the ilium, ischium, and pubis—meet, a deep socket is formed. This is called the acetabulum. Like the shoulder, the hip is a ball-and-socket joint. Unlike the shoulder, the hip is very stable. This joint is so stable that there is actually a suction or vacuum created inside the joint. (This is good news, because hip dislocations are traumatic. Don't worry, though. You will likely never see your son or daughter dislocate a hip.)

The "ball" of the hip joint is the head of the femur (the thighbone). The union of the femur and the acetabulum creates the hip joint, which is surrounded by a thick, tough, ligamentous tissue called the joint capsule. While the joint capsule provides added stability, it also reduces hip motion. In some athletes, the capsule becomes too tight, causing joint restriction. The combination of a deep socket and a thick capsule explains why we cannot move our hips like we can our shoulders.

The thighbone, or femur, supports much of the weight of the body. In fact, femur fractures are rare because the bone is so big. The head of the femur fits in the socket to create the hip joint, as we just learned. The muscles of the thigh help secure the femur to the pelvis. One end of the muscle group attaches to the pelvis and the other end attaches to the femur.

The hip flexors are located in the front of the thigh. When this muscle group contracts, the leg lifts. This motion is called hip flexion. The iliopsoas *(ilio-SO-us)* is a very important hip flexor and is often injured, despite its size. Soccer players, for example, frequently injure this muscle.

The adductors, located on the inside of the thigh, pull the thigh in. This motion is called adduction. The adductors are also called groin muscles, because they are located in the groin area. Hockey players often injure this muscle group. In sports where the athlete stands on one foot while the other leg moves—such as in dance or gymnastics—the adductors stabilize the leg.

The abductors, located on the outside of the hip, pull the leg or thigh away from the body. This motion is called abduction. The gluteus medius, one of the muscles in the buttocks, is the primary abductor.

Located in the back of the thigh, the extensors extend the thigh. The hamstring muscles and the gluteus maximus—the most prominent muscle in the buttocks—are extensor muscles.

Three bursae in the hip are important when it comes to pelvis, hip, and thigh injuries. Remember, bursae are small, fluid-filled sacs that prevent or reduce friction. They are similar to other bursae in the body, and, like other bursae, can be injured during activity.

Hip and Pelvis Injuries

Athletes who frequently move from side to side (like tennis players and basketball players) may inflame or injure the tendon that attaches the gluteus medius muscle to the pelvis. Although this injury can happen because of trauma, it is most often a chronic injury. Your son may complain of a pain in his hip. This pain, like most tendonitis injuries, gradually gets worsen. Gluteus medius tendonitis causes pain along the outside and top of the pelvis. If you suspect gluteus medius tendonitis, ask your son to lay on the floor, on his uninjured side. Tell him to make an imaginary line between his ear, shoulder, hip, knee, and foot. This forces his body to straighten. Then ask him to lift his injured leg, while you push down against his force. If he complains of pain or has weakness, you might suspect a gluteus medius injury.

Treatment of gluteus medius tendonitis is simple: provide ice and relative rest from those activities that cause pain. Anti-inflammatory medications like Advil also work, but always ask your doctor if this is appropriate. Relative rest, again, does not mean inactivity. It means reducing the activities that cause the pain. Once the pain goes away, ask a physical therapist or athletic trainer for specific exercises to strengthen this area. Strengthening the muscle and tendon group often prevents further or recurrent injury.

Athletes may injure other tendons that attach to the pelvis as well, such as the rectus femoris. This tendon attaches near the front of the pelvis. When inflamed, it causes pain when athletes take a shot in soccer or attempt a field goal in football. Again, tendonitis injuries require ice and relative rest, followed by stretching and strengthening exercises. Ask your doctor to refer you to an athletic trainer or physical therapist who will answer specific questions about your child's injury.

A "hip pointer" is a contusion or bruise to the pelvis. This usually occurs in the front of the pelvis where the bone is most prominent. Hockey players often injure this area because they constantly collide with opponents and/or the boards. Football players are at risk for this injury, too. Being tackled, especially if the helmet strikes the pelvis, is a very common cause of hip pointers. At first, the injury may be swollen and painful. Your child may also have problems standing upright, due to pain and muscle spasms. Apply ice to the injury as soon as possible to decrease the pain and spasms. Most importantly, try to remain level-headed about these injuries. They usually look worse than they are, and most athletes feel an improvement after ten to fifteen minutes of ice and rest. Of course, if your child shows no sign of improvement, seek the help of a physician.

Once the pain, swelling, and muscle spasms subside, gently stretch the area. Your child may begin strengthening exercises shortly thereafter to regain the strength he or she lost while the injury was painful. When pain free (or nearly pain free), your child is safe to resume athletic activity. You may find that additional padding will prevent reinjury. Ask your child's coach or an athletic trainer for padding suggestions. Simple foam works very well.

Bursitis

There are three primary bursae in the hip and pelvis. The ischial bursa is near the ischial tuberosity (also known as the "butt bone"). Because of its location, athletes involved in rowing and cycling sports are at risk for bursitis in this area. They may experience pain in the buttocks, especially when sitting. The trochanteric bursa is located along the side of the leg, right where you feel the hip's ball-and-socket joint. Runners are at particular risk for injury to the trochanteric bursa. Iliotibial band (IT band) tightness also contributes to this injury. You may remember ITB syndrome from the Knee chapter. Tightness in the IT band can cause pain in the knee or hip, so stretching this tissue often helps tremendously with trochanteric bursitis. The psoas (pronounced *SO-us)* bursa is deep inside the hip. Athletes with bursitis in that location feel pain deep inside the hip, especially near the front. The psoas muscle is a hip flexor, so hip flexion sometimes causes pain when people have this injury.

Treatment of bursitis injuries is almost always the same. Your child should ice the injury several times per day, refrain from activities that cause pain, and stretch tight muscles, especially the hip flexors and IT band. You should ask your doctor about any hip or pelvis pain that doesn't seem to improve with these simple treatment techniques, especially if it lasts more than a week or two. An athletic trainer may also recommend suggestions for treatment.

Thigh Injuries

Hamstring and Quadriceps Strain

The hamstrings are the muscles in the back of the thigh that extend the hip and bend the leg at the knee. The quadriceps (or quad) is a group of four muscles in the front of the thigh that straightens the leg at the knee. One of these muscles also flexes the hip, lifting the thigh toward the ceiling. These thigh muscles are very important for runners, jumpers, and other athletes.

Many thigh injuries occur when people either stretch incorrectly or overwork the muscles. Injuries also occur during activities that require a sudden, powerful muscle contraction—like when a sprinter explodes out of the starting block or a soccer player attempts a difficult shot. Thigh injuries range in severity from slight pulls to complete ruptures. The symptoms will vary depending on the severity. Mild to moderate muscle strains are common—you can expect your volleyball-playing daughter or basketball-playing son to suffer this type of injury at some point. Minor muscle strains hurt, but they are easy to manage, and most athletes get better very quickly. To treat sore muscles and minor muscle strains, see pages 141 and 142.

Severe muscle strains require immediate medical attention. Any time you notice a deformity, like a divot in the muscle, get the athlete to a physician quickly. A deformity could indicate that the muscle has completely ruptured. Swelling, discoloration, and spasms will also accompany the deformity. Because muscles are filled with blood vessels, severe muscle injuries bleed and cause a lot of swelling. Spasms occur to prevent the athlete from doing more damage to the muscle, acting as a kind of natural splint.

When a muscle completely ruptures, the athlete will feel a snap, pop, or tear. These injuries hurt. If your son mentions that he heard a "pop" and has deformity, he has probably torn a muscle. Managing muscle ruptures correctly is important—you'll want to seek the advice of a physician, and probably a physical therapist or athletic trainer, as well.

In theory, if a muscle ruptures, the athlete should not be able to use it. However, the uninjured muscles will try to "fill in" for the injured one. In any case, you will notice a significant loss of function. Determining whether the loss of function is related to serious muscle injury or simple fear can be tricky. Parents know their children best—if you suspect that your child is significantly limited because of a serious muscle injury, seek medical attention. If you do not notice a muscle deformity or loss of function, you may want to wait a day to see how the injury responds to basic treatment techniques, which we will discuss shortly.

Athletes with a muscle rupture cannot participate in their sport. Not only will they experience too much pain, but their bodies may not allow them to function. Athletes with minor muscle strains, however, may participate if they are functional. Imagine that your daughter wants to play in her basketball tournament, but she has a sore quadriceps. She can do her basketball drills with only mild discomfort. As a parent, you could let her play. Her body will tell her when she has done too much (her quads will hurt a lot). On the other hand, let's imagine that your daughter is quite sore in the quadriceps. You notice that she walks with a limp and she can't really jump very high. As a parent, you should not let her play.

Karl wanted to play in a soccer game, and his injury was very similar to the injury in this last scenario. However, Karl elected to play in the game. The next day, he could barely use his leg, and he missed three weeks of soccer practice while his leg healed. Nate's injury, on the other hand, was similar to the injury in our first hypothetical scenario. He, too, played in his soccer game. The next day, Nate's leg was sore, but no worse. The difference between the two cases was this: prior to the soccer game, Karl had problems walking and doing daily activities, while Nate did not. If your son or daughter can't do normal activities without pain, you shouldn't let him or her participate in an athletic activity until the leg heals.

Groin Strain

Also called "adductor strains," groin strains can vary in severity. The symptoms are similar to quadriceps and hamstring strains. Hockey players are especially susceptible to groin strains. They use their adductors, or groin muscles, a lot, since they pull their legs in after each stride while skating. Tennis players also use their groin muscles when they run the baseline in tennis.

Unlike a quad or hamstring strain, a groin strain can sometimes feel like another injury, such as a hernia. For this reason, many boys and young men feel somewhat shy about telling anyone about it. A groin strain can also feel like a hip flexor strain. Hip flexor strains cause pain when the athlete pulls the thigh up toward the head. A groin strain causes pain when the athlete draws the leg toward the middle of the body. Be certain to have a physician or other medical professional evaluate any groin pain.

If you suspect a complete rupture, seek help immediately. (Although the physician may not "fix" the problem, he or she can provide pain medication.) For sore muscles and mild muscle strains, apply RICE. Ice reduces swelling and spasms, and it controls bleeding within the muscle. It does a great job of reducing pain, too. When your daughter is finished icing her injury, wrap her thigh with an ACE bandage. This reduces swelling and provides some support. Encourage her to gently stretch the muscles. The key to a quick recovery is to maintain muscle length. Don't allow a muscle injury to shorten or tighten the muscle. This may lead not only to more injury, but also decreased performance. Encourage your daughter to do her stretches. She will thank you for it later. Also, avoid pain-causing activity. The purpose of this is twofold: First, these muscles need time to heal. If your daughter never gives her body a chance to heal, it probably won't. Second, when other muscles compensate for the injured muscle, they can become overworked, which leads to injury.

Quadriceps Contusion

Quadriceps contusions are uncommon in noncollision sports. Football, hockey, and soccer players are at risk for these injuries. Although we consider a quad contusion a "bruise," these injuries can be very painful and can drastically cut into performance. If an opponent kicks your soccer-playing child in the thigh, don't just dismiss the injury as insignificant. While many quad contusions are minor and do not cause too much pain, some will hurt a great deal. Managing these injuries right away will reduce problems down the road.

John played high-school basketball. While he was setting a pick, his opponent's knee struck him in the quad. Although it hurt, he didn't tell anyone about it and resumed the game. After the game, he did what most high-school guys do on a Friday night—he went out with his friends. When he woke up the next day, he could barely move his leg. Walking up and down stairs was extremely painful and difficult. Had John managed the injury correctly, he may have prevented these problems.

The best indicator of a quad contusion is the history. Was the athlete kicked or struck by an opponent's knee or helmet, or did the athlete fall on a hard object, striking his or her quad? If the answer is yes to either of these questions, chances are that the athlete has a quad contusion. Other symptoms include pain, swelling, and discoloration. The injury may appear deformed because of swelling or extensive abrasion.

In the absence of deformity and extreme pain, use ice to reduce swelling and control the pain. (Refer to the Evaluation, Treatment, and Prevention chapter.) Ice the area every one to two hours. Next, encourage gentle stretching to improve range of motion and reduce the chance that the injury will limit movement the next day. Sometimes an injury will appear insignificant at the time, then the athlete will wake up the next day to find that he or she can't move the leg. Gentle stretching not only reduces this possibility, it decreases the likelihood that the injury will become more serious or limiting.

An ACE wrap will provide enough compression to reduce swelling. A Neoprene sleeve may also help. Most major sporting goods stores should have Neoprene sleeves available. These sleeves are more costly, but they work well for the more serious cases or when the ACE wrap doesn't provide enough relief.

If you treat the injury in this manner, the quad contusion should heal within two weeks. However, always address any concerns you may have with a medical provider. In serious cases, a condition known as myositis ossificans can develop if the injury is not treated properly or evaluated in time. Myositis ossificans is a condition in which the blood that pools inside an injured muscle calcifies (turns into a bony growth) inside the muscle. This will cause many problems for the patient. Although it doesn't happen that often—and it certainly doesn't happen immediately—a medical provider can advise you if you are concerned about it. Again, this only happens in the most serious cases, but be suspicious of any quad contusion that takes longer than ten to fourteen days to improve.

Femoral Fractures

Although they are very uncommon, femur fractures do occur. Because the femur (thighbone) is so big, you will likely never see one of these injuries; however, you should know what to look for in case it occurs.

Femur fractures can happen anywhere on the femur, but most require significant trauma (like being tackled or struck). Some people fracture the condyles, the pieces of the femur on the sides, near the knee. Other people fracture the neck of the femur, near the hip. Perhaps even more serious are fractures in the middle of the femur. These injuries pose serious problems because of the blood vessels and nerves in the area. Because the femur is so large, fractures are rare in young, otherwise healthy, athletes. We know of one young boy, however, who has brittle bone disease—his femur fractures without any trauma. His case is not the norm, and you would know before long if your child has a condition like this.

You can usually tell the difference between a thigh contusion and a femur fracture. Femur fractures cause visual deformity and excruciating pain. Standing on a femur fracture is terribly painful and could potentially cause more damage. Thigh contusions, on the other hand, are not as painful. If you suspect a femur fracture, don't move or touch the leg—call an ambulance immediately.

Tendon Ruptures

The quadriceps tendon—or patellar tendon—can tear like any other tendon. President Clinton tore his quadriceps tendon stumbling down the stairs. This tendon is responsible for straightening the knee. People in high-contact or collision sports are at the greatest risk for quadriceps and patellar tendon ruptures. Twisting, falling, and quick, explosive movements can cause these injuries. Because the tendon is big (you can feel your tendon just above and below your kneecap), complete rupture is uncommon, especially in children. If the tendon is torn, you or your child will know. The athlete will hear a "pop," feel a snap, and may even see a deformity. If your child describes any of these, seek the help of a physician immediately. In the meantime, ice and immobilize the injury on the way to the doctor.

Conclusion

Injuries to the pelvis, hip, and thigh are quite common in athletics. These injuries can be acute (resulting from excessive force, contact, or collision), or they can be chronic (ongoing stress that causes injury). In either case, your ability to recognize the difference between the two will ultimately tell you when you need emergency care and when you can treat the injury at home.

Injuries can happen to any of the three bones that make up the pelvis. Because the pelvis forms the link between the spine and the lower extremities, injuries to the pelvis can affect activities like walking and running. They can also affect activities like standing upright and sitting in a chair. Obviously, they can affect many different sporting activities.

The muscles that act on the thigh start at the pelvis. Weakness or tightness in one thigh muscle can cause problems with another. For example, tight hip flexors can cause back pain. Tight hamstring muscles can also cause back pain. Indeed, the anatomy is very complex, and there is no way we could highlight every muscle injury to the hip, pelvis, and thigh. Nevertheless, you should realize that muscle weakness or injury to the pelvis area could cause a "pain in the butt!"

Determining the cause of the problem is a job for your healthcare provider. However, if you learn the red flags, your ability to make good decisions will greatly improve. For example, hip pain that gradually becomes worse over time is most likely an overuse injury, such as tendonitis or bursitis. An injury that happens because of a collision with an opponent (or the ground) may be more serious. Chronic injuries can be serious, but they rarely require a trip to the emergency room or urgent care facility, like acute injuries sometimes do.

Frequently Asked Questions

Q: *My son has pain on the outside of his leg near the hip. It's been there for a while. What is it, and do I need to see a physician right away?*

A: It is most likely a bursitis injury. Bursa sacs are tiny sacs that protect muscles and tendons from friction and other injury. However, they can become inflamed. When they do, the pain gradually becomes worse.

Yes, your son should see a physician for this. Your pediatrician or family physician will likely take x-rays to make sure nothing else is causing the pain. This is not an emergency, so you can schedule the appointment for a convenient time.

Q: *My daughter has a pain in the front of her leg. Any suggestions?*

A: Without knowing how the injury happened, we could only suspect that this is a quadriceps muscle strain. The quad is a group of four muscles in the front of the thigh. Athletes who use their legs a lot are at risk for this injury. If the injury happened as a result of a collision (like in hockey), we would be more likely to suspect a serious injury.

Tell your daughter to stretch well before activity and to ice her leg after activity. Also, ask that she refrain from the activities that cause her pain. She may still participate in other activities that do not cause discomfort. If her condition does not improve within a few days, ask your healthcare provider for advice.

Q: *My daughter's hips appear uneven. Is this serious?*

A: It could be. Uneven hips could indicate scoliosis, an abnormal curvature in the spine. This condition affects girls more than boys, and the effects vary depending on the severity of the curve. If you notice that your daughter has uneven hips, call your doctor. Your daughter will need an x-ray.

Sometimes the hips can be out of alignment because of muscle tightness or injury, although this is more difficult to see with the untrained eye. In any case, contact your healthcare provider for an evaluation. Unless this is the result of a collision (and causes a lot of pain), this is not an emergency. Feel free to make the appointment when it's convenient for you.

Q: *Is it possible for a child to fracture a hip? I thought only old people did this.*

A: While it is possible for a young child to fracture a hip, it is not likely. Hip fractures are far more common among older people. Your child is more likely to develop a stress fracture in the femur from an overuse injury, or fracture the femur following a twisting or collision force. Femur fractures are painful and require immediate attention.

Another kind of fracture is an avulsion fracture. This is where the muscle tears itself from the bone, taking a chunk of the bone with it. This does happen to children, and it is incredibly painful. Avulsion fractures happen following explosive bursts of activity, like sprinting or jumping. Athletes hear a "pop" and feel a snap.

If your child has these symptoms, seek help immediately.

Q: *Are most hip or pelvis injuries muscle related?*

A: Many injuries are muscle or tendon related. Many are injuries to the bursae. In the absence of acute injury (like in contact sports), fractures are unlikely. Even stress fractures take time to develop. Therefore, most injuries respond well to RICE. Gentle stretching and light strengthening exercises often prevent reinjury.

Contributing Author: Lorie Schleck, PT

Lorie is a physical therapist with the Institute for Athletic Medicine, Robbinsdale Clinic, where she specializes in lower extremity injuries, especially as they pertain to running injuries. Lorie has coordinated the IAM Running Program and she currently edits the SidelineView, *a publication regarding various topics in sports medicine that is distributed to people throughout the country. Lorie teaches a course on hip and pelvis injuries and rehabilitation throughout the country. Lorie and her husband, Jim, have one child, Ben.*

Contributing Author: Reneé Ledin, MS, ATC/R

Reneé is a certified athletic trainer with the Institute for Athletic Medicine, Burnsville Clinic. She is also the Head Athletic Trainer for Burnsville High School. She has held both of these positions since 1991. Reneé is very active in the National Athletic Trainers' Association Board of Certification, as she is one of six members appointed to the Credentialing Committee.

Contributing Author: Brenda Dolejs, ATC/R

Brenda is a certified athletic trainer with the Institute for Athletic Medicine, Apple Valley Clinic. She is also the Head Athletic Trainer for Apple Valley High School, where she provides athletic training services to over 1,500 athletes. Brenda is active in the HealthClub Referral Program at the Institute for Athletic Medicine. Brenda and her husband, Chris, recently had their first child, Collin.

Chapter 9

The Spine

For many people, back and neck injuries conjure up devastating images, like the tragedy with Christopher Reeves. In reality, most back and neck injuries do not require surgery, and many get better within a few weeks. Exceptions, however, certainly exist. This chapter will highlight some of the different injuries that affect the spine. We will also discuss simple ways for parents and coaches to recognize the difference between a serious medical emergency, and a back or neck pain that does not require a visit to the emergency room.

Anatomy and Biomechanics

Understanding the simple structure of the spine will help you recognize the serious injuries that could affect it. The spine is a series of small bones, called vertebrae, that join to protect the spinal cord. The spinal cord is the big nerve tissue that carries information from the brain to the rest of body—kind of like an "information superhighway." Information travels from the brain to tissues throughout the body, and information from the tissues goes to the brain through the spinal cord. Some of the transfer of information is involuntary—we don't consciously make the decision to breathe, for example. However, we do need to tell our muscles to work during activity. This occurs because of the spinal cord.

The spine is made up of vertebrae, discs, ligaments, muscles, and tendons. There are four types of vertebrae—the cervical vertebrae, the thoracic vertebrae, the lumbar vertebrae, and the sacrum (five bones fused into one). Seven cervical vertebrae protect the spinal cord near the neck. Because these vertebrae only need to support the weight of the head, they are the smallest of the three types of vertebrae. Twelve thoracic vertebrae protect the spinal cord in the middle of the back. They also serve as an attachment point for the ribs. These vertebrae are larger than the cervical vertebrae, and they increase in size as they go down the spine. The lumbar vertebrae support much of the weight of the body, so they are the biggest of all. Typically, there are five lumbar vertebrae, although some people are born with six. (This is not a problem.) The lumbar vertebrae protect the spinal cord near the low back.

Spine (viewed from the left side)

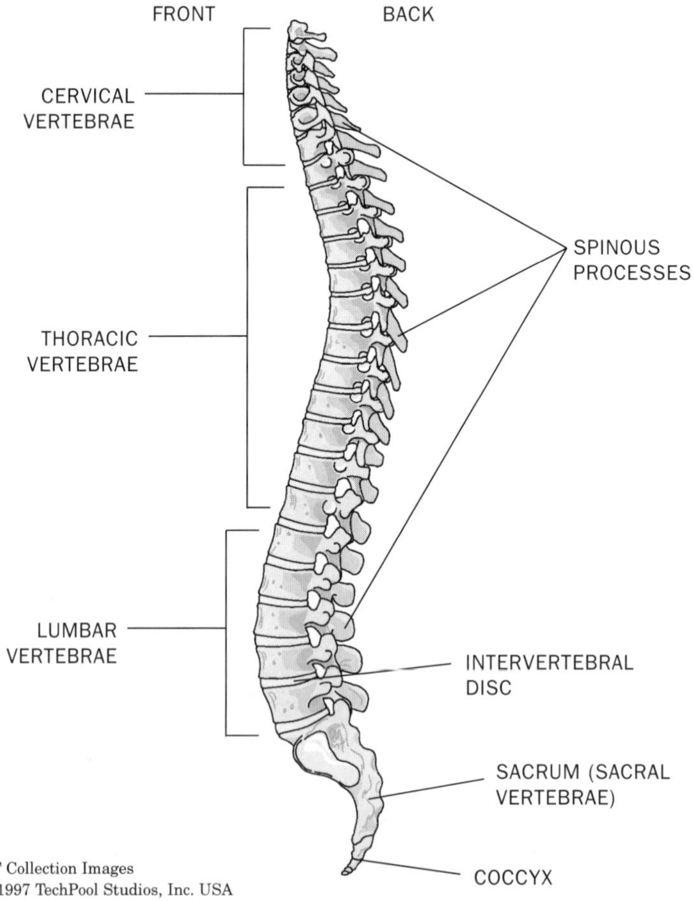

The vertebrae themselves have many different parts; however, only some of the parts will influence your evaluation of an injury. The body of the vertebra, which is the largest portion, supports weight. It also gives structure and form to our spine. The spinous processes are the little bumps you can feel on your back and neck. Muscles and tendons attach to these. Each vertebra also has a transverse process—another, less detectable, portion of the bone—to which muscles and tendons also attach. Finally, the vertebral foramen (the plural is foramina) is the hole through which the spinal cord passes. Some people have narrow foramina, which can put pressure on the spinal cord.

Where each of the vertebrae lock together, they form joints. Ligaments—the tissues that connect bone to bone—hold the vertebrae together. Many people do not know that you can sprain the joints of your back much like you can sprain your ankle joint or knee joint. Excessive twisting, like in gymnastics, can sprain the ligaments that connect the spine.

Vertebrae and Spinal Cord

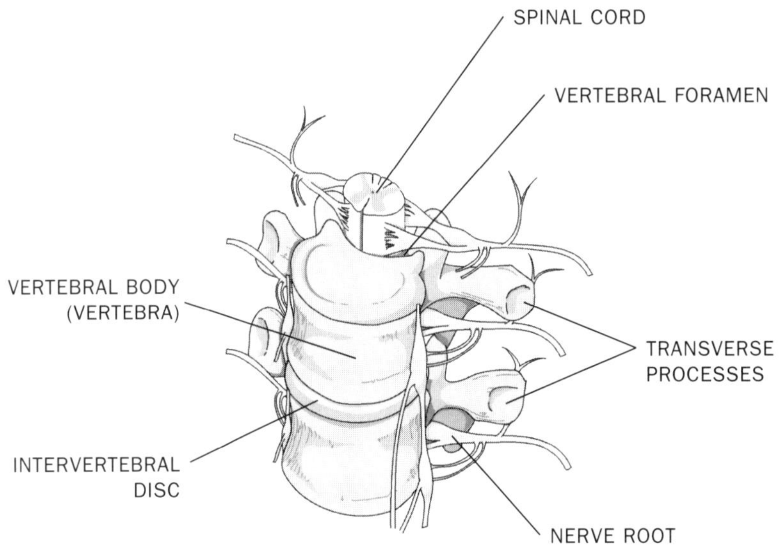

Between the vertebrae rest small discs that help cushion the spine when we are active. These discs can become damaged. Think of the discs as jelly doughnuts. The outside of the disc is somewhat more firm than the inside. Inside the disc is a substance like the jelly in a jelly doughnut.

The sacrum, a wedge-shaped bone, is located just below the lumbar vertebrae and consists of five fused vertebrae. The sacrum connects with the pelvis. Injuries to the pelvis and sacrum can cause low back pain. Likewise, injury to the low back can affect the pelvis and sacrum. On the pelvis, the bones we call our "butt bones" (the ones that get sore if we sit too long) serve as attachments to the hamstring muscles (muscles in the back of the thigh). The tailbone (coccyx) is the small bone that hurts like crazy if you slip on the ice and, as my little sister Becky describes, "fall on your caboose."

Muscles and tendons also attach to the vertebrae, so muscle and tendon strain can cause back pain, too. For example, the scalene muscles originate on the transverse processes of the cervical vertebrae. They insert on the upper two ribs. Designed to flex and rotate the neck (as well as assist in inhalation), these muscles, when injured, cause pain with neck flexion and rotation. On the other hand, injury to the intertransversarii muscles around the vertebrae makes it hard for people to bend from one side to the other.

The spine is unique. It has the ability to rotate, flex and extend (bend forward and backward), and bend from side to side. Because of the small joints in the spine, we have the ability to move extensively. However, because of this ability, we risk overuse injuries. Doing the same repetitive task over a long period of time, such as lifting improperly, can cause back injury and pain. Trauma and poor posture can cause back injury as well.

Cervical Spine and Neck Injuries

The neck is a complex series of joints. The seven cervical vertebrae allow us to look up and down, rotate our head, and move our head from side to side. We have a great deal of motion in our neck, and this motion is imperative in athletics. Athletes are at risk for injury when they cannot see their opponents around them. For example,

Justin, a football player, had a neck strain that prevented him from turning his head from side to side. He could not look over his shoulders to see where his tacklers were. This injury severely compromised his ability to protect himself. The coaches and the athletic trainer decided that it was in his best interest to miss a game for injury reasons.

Only the most severe neck injuries can lead to permanent paralysis and death. Medicine has made such incredible strides that many accident victims, who were once thought to be destined to life in a wheelchair, can now walk and live normal lives. But, indeed, many people with spinal cord injuries in the neck area never walk again. Many never feed themselves or even breathe for themselves. Consequently, managing a neck injury can be one of the most important things you can ever learn as a parent or coach. One mistake can come at a great cost.

We discussed the first-aid treatment of neck injuries in the Emergency Procedures chapter. Here we will highlight the major points. The vast majority of serious neck injuries occur when an athlete strikes another player or an immovable object with great force. For example, football players are at risk when they make contact, especially if they do not keep their head up when they tackle or are tackled. Hockey players are at risk if they get checked into the boards from behind. Gymnasts and divers are at risk if they fall incorrectly on their heads.

If you notice any of the following red flags, call 911 immediately. Even moving the athlete can cause great harm.

- Pain on the "bumps" in the back of the neck. This could indicate a vertebral injury. Without an x-ray, you cannot be certain that there is no fracture. Fractured bones are unstable, which can lead to spinal cord injury. Moving an unstable neck is not good.

- Referred pain down the arm and into the elbow and/or fingers. Referred pain could indicate several different injuries; however, physicians often require x-rays or CT scans to know if the spinal cord was damaged.

- Numbness into the arm or hand that does not improve within a few seconds. Remember that the spinal cord carries information from the brain to the the arm and hand (and from the hand and arm to the brain). If the cord is damaged, the information has no way to get from point A to point B. Information cannot travel on a nerve pathway if the nerve is damaged. Another possible cause for the tingling or numbness is a peripheral nerve injury (an injury to the nerves traveling down the arm), but your primary concern is to treat it as a serious spinal cord injury.
- Loss of strength. Have the athlete squeeze your fingers and move his or her feet. If the child cannot squeeze your fingers or move his or her toes, be suspicious. Lack of strength is a good indicator of serious injury, especially if other red flags are present.
- Unconsciousness. If the athlete is unable to communicate with you, assume the worst. Never, ever, dismiss a neck injury because the play did not look too serious. If the athlete is unable to tell you how his or her neck feels, treat it like a serious neck injury. Allow more qualified medical personnel to handle the situation. Contact 911 and monitor the athlete's ABCs.

Stingers

The terms "stingers" and "burners" are used interchangeably. They refer to an injury to the brachial plexus nerve complex. This nerve complex reaches from the spinal cord in the neck down the shoulder, sending information from the nerves in the neck to the arm. All nerve injuries must be evaluated by a physician. When an athlete suffers multiple stingers, long-term complications become more likely.

While athletes who participate in contact sports are the most likely to get stingers, football players seem to be at a particular risk. The big question for youth coaches and parents is how to tell the difference between a stinger and a more serious neck injury.

Stingers have the following signs and symptoms:

- Radiating pain down the arm. This often feels like you hit the "funny bone" in your elbow.
- Tingling or burning into the fingers.
- Poor strength and/or an inability to raise or lower the arm.
- Pain into the shoulder and muscles of the neck.

With stingers, these symptoms get better within a few seconds or minutes. Serious neck injuries, on the other hand, do not get better.

Most stingers do not cause serious systemic complications. In other words, the body does not go into protection mode, lowering blood pressure and shutting down vital organs. In true spinal cord injuries, however, the body sometimes shuts down these systems in order to protect the heart and the brain.

One football player, Craig, had stingers for a full year before he told his athletic trainer about the problem. He simply assumed that stingers were normal and that they were not significant, since the symptoms always got better within a few seconds. When his athletic trainer referred him to a physician, the results were shocking. Craig was missing a portion of the (fourth) cervical vertebra. In effect, his neck was not able to protect his spinal cord from injury in football. The stingers Craig had were an indication of a larger problem.

Luckily, Craig did not have a serious neck injury. But he could have. Because of his condition, Craig quit football. He could not be certain that another hit or another stinger would not cause more harm. Craig will lead a normal life and be able to do just about everything he wants to. However, he will not be able to participate in contact sports. Craig's case highlights the importance of having a physician evaluate all neck injuries.

A question that some parents may have is, "Now that I know it's a stinger, what do I do about it?" Follow these guidelines:

- Never allow a player to return to the game unless a physician or athletic trainer has cleared him or her. Medical professionals can assess all nerve levels to make certain that the nerves supplying information to the rest of the arm are working properly.

- Teach proper technique. Tackling with the head down is an invitation for disaster. Proper technique can prevent many of these neck injuries.
- Fit your players with the proper equipment. Football players with stingers may find relief with a neck roll or other padding that limits excessive neck motion.
- Consult with an athletic trainer or physical therapist who can recommend some strengthening exercises. Strengthening the muscles of the neck and shoulder will help prevent these injuries.

Muscle Strains

Muscle injuries can happen in the neck just as they can happen in the leg or arm. If you have ever had a muscle spasm in your neck, you know they are serious. When we injure our muscles, the body reacts to protect itself. Muscles spasm to protect and prevent further injury. But this spasm is what causes pain and immobility.

Most neck strains cause pain and limit motion. Stretching the muscle in spasm hurts. If the muscle on the left side of your daughter's neck is in spasm, it will hurt for her to put her right ear to her right shoulder. Putting her chin to her chest, however, may not cause as much pain. In some cases, all motion causes pain.

Muscle strains typically cause pain to one side of the neck or the other. With muscle strains, however, the primary pain is *not* on the spinous processes (the little "bumps" in the neck that attach the muscles to the spine). If these bumps hurt, consult your physician immediately.

Muscle strains and spasms heal more quickly than disc, ligament, or bone injuries do. Muscles have a large blood supply, which means the body has the ability to heal itself efficiently. In addition, these injuries respond well to treatment.

Treating neck strains is similar to treating other injuries. Keep in mind the following:

- Rest and ice the neck (RICE doesn't quite apply here, since it's hard to compress and elevate a neck injury). Along with antibiotics and vaccines, rest and ice are treatments that will have the greatest impact on health over time. They work wonders, especially to reduce muscle spasms and control pain.
- Encourage pain-free range of motion. Maintaining the athlete's range of motion will speed his or her recovery. This is not to suggest that you should make your son do neck circles if it causes pain; rather, he should maintain whatever range of motion he can. Slowly, but surely, the range will improve and the muscle spasms will go away. In addition, you may wish to consult with a physical therapist or athletic trainer regarding specific stretches and exercises for your child's specific injury.
- Allow participation in sports only if the injury does not pose a safety risk, as we discussed earlier. For example, if your daughter plays goalie in hockey, she needs to be able to turn her head quickly. If she cannot do this, her play suffers (which also affects the team) and she risks additional injury.

Thoracic Spine Injuries

The thoracic spine has twelve vertebrae that form the middle of the back. Ribs attach to these vertebrae, as do muscles that perform many different functions. For example, the rhomboids originate on the little bumps (the spinous processes) in the thoracic spine and attach to the scapula (the shoulder blade). The function of the rhomboids is to pull the scapula toward the spine and stabilize it during throwing activity. Therefore, even activities that do not appear to involve the muscles of the spine may cause mid-back pain.

Muscle Strains

Most injuries to the thoracic spine are muscle related. Injuries to the trapezius muscles (the big muscles on either side of the neck, between the neck and upper shoulder) are common, especially among school-age children. Children frequently have poor posture, and poor posture creates muscle strain. Muscle strain may also result from injuries such as whiplash, forceful contact (when being tackled, for example), and overuse.

Muscle strains in the back are similar to muscle strains in other parts of the body. Certain activities cause pain, including stretching. Muscle strains usually take about five to seven days to heal properly, especially if the patient is correcting the cause of the strain. If a child improves his or her posture, for example, muscle strain may disappear. In fact, sitting up straight and keeping the shoulders back will go a long way toward improving the health of the entire back, not just the thoracic area.

Scoliosis

Scoliosis is a condition common to many young children—as many as 10 percent. In fact, most schools screen their students for this condition. Scoliosis is a curvature of the spine. When you look at a child with scoliosis, you may notice one shoulder lower than the other or one hip higher than the other. Mild forms of this condition affect both boys and girls between ten and fifteen years old. The more severe cases, however, seem to afflict girls more often. While many children will grow out of this condition naturally, others may require specific exercises or a brace. Few cases actually require surgery.

The key to treating scoliosis is to recognize the symptoms early on. While scoliosis can be easily diagnosed with an x-ray, there are other ways to detect scoliosis without your child even knowing. Examine full body pictures. Are your daughter's shoulders level? Do her hips appear level? Look at your son's back while he swims or plays at the beach. Scoliosis will cause a curve that may be visible. You might notice that the muscles on one side of his back are more developed than those on the other side. Examine your child's clothing. Your daughter's pants may not seem to fit quite right. If her pant legs appear to be different lengths, it could be that her hips are unequal—another sign of scoliosis. If you recognize any of these signs or have any questions regarding scoliosis, consult your physician.

Internal Organ Injury

Not all back pain is caused from ligament, tendon, disc, or bone injury. Some thoracic pain may be linked to internal organ injury. Kidney stones are a good example; they can cause constant pain to the low or mid back. The same is true with aneurysms. (An aneurysm is a weakening of the artery wall, which, if left untreated, can lead to extreme blood loss and even death.) These, too, can cause back pain. For that reason, if you or your family member complains of back pain that does not respond to any treatment, consult your physician. Fortunately, the above diagnoses are not common in children or adolescents. Your teenage daughter probably won't pass a kidney stone or have an aneurysm.

Lumbar Spine and Low Back Injuries

People of all ages injure their low backs. The good news is that over 75 percent of all back injuries do not require surgery. Most get better with conservative treatment—physical therapy, medication, exercise, behavior modification, and rest. However, there are situations in which conservative treatments fail and surgery is necessary. As with other injuries, the key to treating low back injuries is to prevent them.

There are several steps your athlete can take to prevent injuries to his or her low back:

- Emphasize good posture. Maintaining a slight curve in your low back is very important. Avoid working in a hunched position. Sitting stooped over a desk—especially for prolonged periods of time—can place a lot of stress on the ligaments, discs, and other soft-tissue structures of the low back.
- Encourage your children to lift correctly. We have all heard the phrase, "Lift with your legs, not with your back." There is a lot of truth to this. Bending over to lift

objects of any weight increases stress on the low back, which can cause injury.

- Teach young athletes to stay physically fit. Too many Big Macs at McDonald's can add a few pounds to the waistline and more stress to the back. People with higher fitness levels have fewer back injuries.

Spondylolysthesis and Spondylolysis

Spondylolysthesis *(spahn-deh-lo-lehs-THEE-sis)* involves a fracture to a lumbar vertebra, which causes one vertebra to slip forward over the other. This condition can happen because of acute injury, like when your child falls while skiing. It can also happen if a vertebral stress fracture (spondylolysis) is left untreated, causing the vertebra to fracture completely. A few people are born with this condition; some do not experience many problems.

With spondylolysthesis, the fifth lumbar vertebra usually slips forward over the first sacral vertebra. Physicians will call this an L5-S1 slip. The amount of slippage defines the degree of severity, which ranges from I to IV. A Grade-I spondylolysthesis means that the bone has slipped up to 25 percent. A Grade-II means that the bone has slipped between 25 and 50 percent, and so on. Most athletes will not experience a Grade-III or -IV injury. Many people lead active, highly-competitive lives with Grade-I injuries. In fact, they may not even know that they have one. X-rays are required to make this diagnosis.

Spondylolysis *(spahn-deh-LOL-isis)* is a stress fracture in the vertebra. It may be either congenital or the result of over-activity. If left untreated, the stress fracture will fracture completely. Complete fractures lead to unstable joints, resulting in a spondylolysthesis. Many athletes who have low back pain for two to three months have this type of injury. Determining the cause of the stress is critical to preventing further damage.

Gymnasts, divers, and other athletes who bend backward a lot (like when a gymnast does a back handspring on the beam) are more prone to spondylolysis. Even offensive linemen in football sometimes have these injuries, because they are always being blocked into positions where they must bend backward.

To identify spondylolysthesis or spondylolysis, consider the following. Pain is most evident when the person bends backward. Bending forward eases and reduces the pain. People with these injuries often have tight hip flexor muscles (muscles in the front of the hip). The muscles pull the pelvis forward, which increases the curve in the low back. If this curve increases too much, the bones pinch together, causing pain. Patients may also have weak abdominal muscles, which fail to adequately support the back and trunk. Many people find relief from the pain by stretching their hip flexors and strengthening their abdominal muscles.

While some low back injuries are related to muscle spasm and strain, and others are related to ligamentous sprain (overstretched ligaments), athletes with a "spondy" feel intense bone pain. (If touching the small bumps on the low back causes pain, ask your physician if an x-ray would be appropriate.) If the bone has slipped far enough forward, it can place pressure on the spinal nerves. This pressure can cause pain and dysfunction to one or both legs.

Treatment for these injuries involves several components. First, identify the cause of the problem. Poor technique, improper footwear, or weak supporting muscles can cause low back pain. If you are able to identify the cause of the injury, you can take steps to prevent further problems.

Ice low back pain. Ice is important, especially after activity. Like other injuries, ice will reduce spasms, pain, and inflammation. You can use moist heat seventy-two hours after an acute injury. However, because most of these injuries are chronic in nature, remember the rule of thumb—heat before activity, ice after. Also, reduce pain-causing activity. This does not mean that your child should assume bed rest, nor does it mean that he or she cannot play. It simply means that your child should avoid heavy practices and meets until his or her back feels better. In other words, give physical therapy and other medical treatment time to work.

Tell athletes to make therapeutic exercise as much a part of their day as brushing their teeth and washing their face. Strengthening the muscles of the abdomen and stabilizing the low back is also helpful. Physicians, physical therapists, or athletic trainers can suggest easy exercises, but athletes must do these exercises regularly. TV commercials, for example, are a good time to do these exercises.

Disc Injuries

Disc injuries occur when the outer wall of a disc becomes weak. When this happens, the inner portion of the disc bulges (herniates), putting pressure on the spinal cord or nerves.

Lumbar discs can be injured in one of two ways: through acute injuries or chronic injuries. Lifting a heavy object with the wrong technique can cause an acute disc injury.

Disc disease, a process where the disc degenerates and dehydrates, causes chronic problems. Look for the following red flags:

- Pain while bending over. If your son has pain into the buttocks or legs when he bends over to tie his shoes, be concerned. Unlike "spondy" injuries (see pages 160 and 161), disc injuries cause pain while bending forward. Spondy injuries cause pain while bending backward.
- Radiating pain, numbness, or tingling into the buttocks, thigh, lower leg, or feet. This happens when the disc puts pressure on the nerve. Have your child lie on his or her back and lift up his or her leg. If this causes pain (or any other symptoms, such as burning, tingling, or radiating pain), be extra concerned. This is a good indication of a disc injury. In the absence of a traumatic injury, these symptoms require evaluation by a physician in a clinical setting. Your child probably will not need to go to an emergency room. However, if these symptoms appear because of a hard tackle or a fall off the uneven bars, call 911.
- Weakness or poor reflexes. Sometimes, the disc can block the "information superhighway" so that muscles do not receive the signal to work. In these cases, the muscles do not function, despite the athlete's best efforts. Poor reflexes may also indicate nerve damage, possibly the result of a disc injury.

To treat a disc injury, consult a physician. Doctors will often require an MRI or CT scan to identify the specific nature of the disc injury. This information will help define treatment strategies. Trying to evaluate and treat these injuries without the help of a physician can lead to further injury. A physical therapist or athletic trainer who has extensive rehabilitation experience with low back injuries will be able to provide specific exercises for the patient.

Make an effort to identify the patient's sleeping patterns. For example, if your daughter sleeps on her back, instruct her to place a pillow under her knees when she sleeps. This reduces stress to the low back and corresponding discs. If she sleeps on her side, place the pillow between her legs. If she sleeps on her stomach, place the pillow under her pelvis. This reduces low back stress. In addition, ice the low back and avoid poor posture.

Follow the exercise programs given by your physician, physical therapist, or athletic trainer. If your son has a disc problem, strengthening his abdominal (stomach) and gluteal (buttock) muscles will improve his trunk strength and stability. Dedication to an exercise plan separates the people with long-term back pain from those with short-term back pain.

Avoid pain-causing activities. Again, this does not mean complete bed rest. Walking is great exercise, if the athlete's back can tolerate it. If it causes too much pain, limit even this activity. In other words, instruct your son or daughter to do whatever feels comfortable.

Muscle Strains

Muscle strains in the low back may exhibit the same symptoms as muscle strains in the neck (see page 156). The same treatments will apply. Keep in mind, however, that tight hamstrings, quadriceps, and hip flexors can cause low back pain. Stretching these muscles is very important.

The abdominal muscles also affect the low back, as do the gluteal muscles. These muscle groups help stabilize the spine and pelvis during activity. Strengthening these muscles, increasing flexibility, and using correct posture and lifting techniques is good medicine. In fact, these principles may eliminate most back pain.

Frequently Asked Questions

Q: *My son complains of lower back pain after cross-country practice. What can I do to help him?*

A: You should recommend that he ice his sore back after practice, and remind him of the importance of stretching before and after practice. A mild hot pack before practice sometimes will help loosen the tight muscles in his back. Furthermore, over-the-counter medications like Advil help relieve the inflammation that causes pain.

Q: *I don't think my daughter has scoliosis, but some of the little bumps in her spine seem to stick out further than others. Should I be worried?*

A: Probably not. The little bumps are prominent on many people, especially at the base of the neck and upper back. They can be difficult to see, however, in people with a lot of muscle mass or fat tissue in the area. If the bumps cause pain, see a physician.

QUICK REFERENCE TABLE

Symptom	Possible Cause	Action
Sharp neck pain after forceful contact or motor vehicle accident.	Cervical neck fracture and/or spinal cord injury.	Immobilize the athlete and call 911 immediately.
Radiating pain down the arms.	Cervical nerve or disc injury.	In the absence of trauma, see a physician immediately. With trauma, call 911.
Neck pain on either side of the little bumps in the neck.	Muscle strain.	Ice, gently stretch the muscles in the neck, and see a physical therapist, athletic trainer, or physician with your questions.
Stiff neck, with or without spine pain.	Ligament injury, muscle or tendon strain, or cervical vertebrae injury. Some infections can cause neck pain as well.	In the absence of trauma, see above. With trauma, contact your physician immediately.
Mid-back pain, without trauma	Rhomboid or other muscle strain. Poor posture or excessive slouching may cause this.	Ice and stretch. See a physician if this condition does not improve within a few days. Also, pay special attention to posture.
Spine curvature.	Scoliosis.	See a physician for x-rays. This is not an emergency.
Back pain that neither improves nor worsens with stretching.	Referred pain from abdomen (i.e., kidney stone).	See your physician as soon as possible.

(CONTINUES ON NEXT PAGE)

Symptom	Possible Cause	Action
Low back pain that gets worse with bending forward.	Lumbar disc injury or muscle injury.	Ice, stretch, strengthen the abdominal and buttock muscles. See your physician as soon as possible.
Radiating pain down one or both legs.	Disc or lumbar nerve injury, possibly tight lower extremity nerves.	In the absence of trauma, find a comfortable position for rest. See your physician as soon as possible to request physical therapy. With trauma, call 911.
Specific bone pain on the spine that increases when you bend backward.	Spondylolysthesis or spondylolysis.	See your physician for x-rays. Ice and stretch. Request therapy from a physical therapist or athletic trainer.
Sore low back (can't bend over, walk, etc.).	Ligament injury, muscle strain, and/or disc injury. It could also indicate an internal organ injury.	Ice, stretch as tolerated, and see your medical provider. In the absence of trauma, this does not require a 911 call.

Contributing Author: Lori Lebert, MS, ATC/R

Lori is a certified athletic trainer with the Institute for Athletic Medicine, where she supervises a staff of over thirty athletic trainers. She is also the Head Athletic Trainer at Park Center High School, a position she has held for eleven years. Lori served as president of the Minnesota Athletic Trainers' Association and recently received the National Athletic Trainers' Association Service Award for dedicated service to the profession of athletic training. She and her husband, Louis, have three children, Ed, Louis II, and Nicholas.

Contributing Author: Scott Kulstad, MEd, ATC/R

With Appreciation: Lynnelle Gelinske, MPT

Chapter 10

The Shoulder

The shoulder is one of the most fascinating joints in the human body. Because of the shoulder, we can lift a barbell overhead, propel our bodies through water, and throw a baseball. The shoulder can move more than any other joint in the body. However, because the shoulder has so much mobility (range of motion), the potential for injury is always present. People of all ages suffer shoulder injuries. Swimmers and baseball players are particularly susceptible, as are athletes serving in volleyball or tennis. These sports rely on the shoulder to perform specific, often repetitive, activities.

Although we make great demands of the shoulder joint, we can still keep it healthy. By maintaining strength and mobility and by not putting unreasonable stress on the shoulder (by pitching a baseball game without warming up, for example), we can avoid injuries and continue to do the things we enjoy.

Anatomy

Four bones, four joints, and almost thirty muscles make up the shoulder. These structures must work together for the shoulder to function normally. The bony parts of the shoulder are the scapula (shoulder blade)—which includes the acromion process and the glenoid—the clavicle (collarbone), the sternum (chest bone), and the humerus (upper arm bone).

The sternum is very important because it links the shoulder to the rest of the body. The sternum connects to the clavicle. The clavicle runs from the sternum out to the scapula, the largest bone in the joint. The scapula runs along the back of the rib cage. The acromion process, an extension of the scapula, connects to the clavicle.

Right Shoulder (viewed from the front)

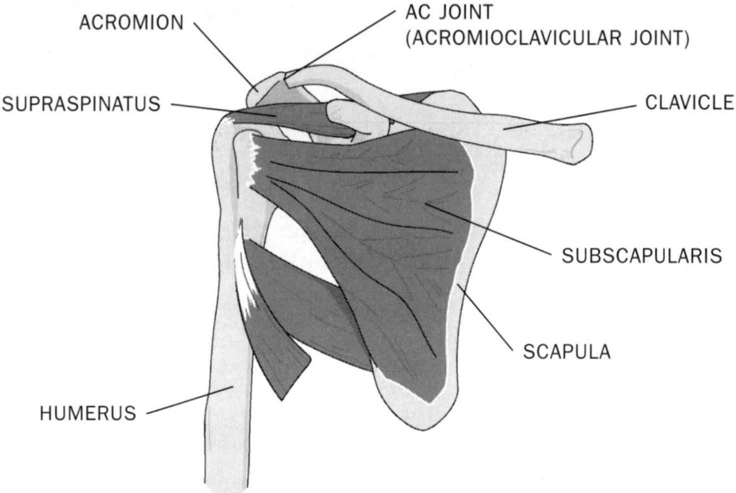

Right Shoulder (viewed from the back)

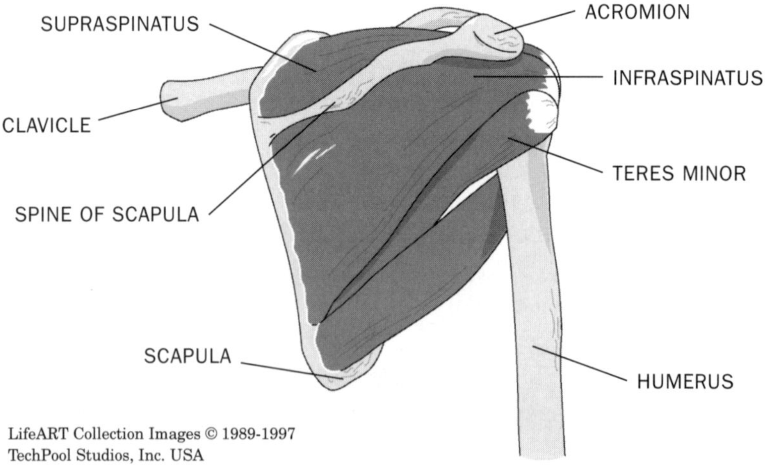

The glenoid is the joint socket. It is actually a part of the scapula, or shoulder blade, but it is inside the shoulder joint, under the acromion process. The acromion process is like the roof over the shoulder joint. The glenoid connects to the humerus (major bone in the upper arm), forming the GH joint (glenohumeral joint), which is the primary shoulder joint. This joint allows us to rotate and move our arm. The glenoid also has a piece of cartilage-like material called a labrum. The glenoid labrum is similar to the meniscus in the knee. It provides some stability to the shoulder. It is, however, a soft tissue and not a bone.

Physical therapists, athletic trainers, and physicians will talk about the four joints in the shoulder. However, we will only discuss the three most critical ones—those that young athletes are most likely to injure. These are the acromioclavicular joint (AC joint), the sternoclavicular joint (SC joint), and glenohumeral joint (GH joint).

The AC joint is where the clavicle and the acromion connect. This joint allows the bones to move forward, backward, up, and down. Ligaments and a joint capsule hold the bones together. Several muscles that attach here keep the joint stable and aid in movement.

The SC joint connects the arm, shoulder blade, and collarbone to the chest bone. This joint does not move very much because ligaments keep it stable. Injuries to this joint can be serious if the collarbone is pushed backward. The lungs are behind the SC joint, and if the joint is damaged, the lungs can be injured as well. Fortunately, this type of injury is not common.

The GH joint is a "ball-and-socket" joint. The ball is the top of the humerus and the socket is the glenoid (remember that the glenoid is a part of the scapula). In this ball and socket joint, the ball is larger than the flat-shaped socket. Unlike the hip—a true ball-and-socket joint—the shoulder more closely resembles a baseball sitting on a golf tee. Muscles, ligaments, and the joint capsule help hold the joint together. The joint capsule is the broad connective tissue that surrounds the joint.

The shoulder muscles cause movement and provide dynamic stability for the GH joint. Dynamic stability is the body's ability to respond to physical activity or stress. It is this stability that helps keep the shoulder joint in place when we are active. The four major stabilizing muscles are the supraspinatus, infraspinatus, teres minor, and subscapularis. (The acronym for these muscles is SITS.) Together, the muscles are called the rotator cuff.

The supraspinatus helps us move the arm up and away from the body. The infraspinatus stabilizes the arm when we are active, and it externally rotates the arm. The teres minor also externally rotates the arm. The subscapularis internally rotates the arm. Another muscle, the biceps brachii, is considered part of the elbow joint, but it also moves and stabilizes the shoulder.

The deltoid muscle (of which there are three parts—an anterior, or front, part; a medial, or middle, part; and the posterior, or back) is the largest muscle in the shoulder. It sits over the shoulder joint. This muscle raises the arm to the front, side, and back. The pectoralis major (commonly called the "pecs") and the latissimus dorsi (commonly called the "lats") also assist in shoulder motions such as swinging a golf club and hitting a tennis ball.

Shoulder Injuries

Shoulder injuries are among the most common injuries we see in physical therapy. People put many different demands on their shoulder, leading to a variety of injuries. Three different patients could have three different shoulder injuries and require three different exercise programs. Athletic activity puts a great deal of stress on the shoulder. The hockey slap shot, football stiff arm, and uneven-bar routine—as well as swimming, weight lifting, swinging a golf club, pitching a baseball, spiking a volleyball, and serving in tennis—all stress the shoulder. Chances are good that your child participates in one of these activities.

Shoulder Impingement

Inflammation in the GH joint is known as shoulder impingement. With this injury, the bursa sac and/or rotator cuff could be inflamed. The most common sign of impingement is pain when reaching the arm overhead, accompanied by loss of strength and/or shoulder motion. Athletes also may have trouble reaching across their body, especially with their arm held chest-high.

With shoulder impingement, the pain gradually worsens over time. It may take anywhere from a few days to a few weeks to notice the pain. However, most people who experience this injury are involved in sports that demand a lot of the shoulder, such as baseball or swimming, and may therefore experience the pain while participating in their sport.

The pain may start as mild soreness after a workout. As the injury progresses, your son may change the way he throws a baseball, for example, to compensate for the pain. Eventually, if the shoulder is left untreated, his performance will suffer as he becomes increasingly unable to control the aim or speed of the throw. At this point, he may be unable to perform at all. Fortunately, most parents don't let their children progress to this point before seeking medical attention.

With shoulder impingement, lying on the affected side is very painful. Even simple, everyday functions become difficult. If your daughter's shoulder is extremely inflamed, she may have trouble putting her hair in a ponytail or brushing her teeth. Although shoulder impingement takes some time to heal, the shoulder should improve with therapy and exercise. Katie, a first-year swimmer, suffered from shoulder impingement. Her shoulder gradually became worse as the season went on. At one point, she could not do many of her daily activities without pain. Katie ended up having to miss the last half of her season while her shoulder recovered.

The causes for shoulder impingement vary from person to person. However, most people suffer this injury because of one or more of the following reasons:

- Shoulder instability. In an unstable shoulder, the rotator cuff muscles fail to stabilize the "ball" on the "tee." In other words, the head of the humerus moves excessively on the glenoid (the socket). This movement inflames the soft tissues in the joint.
- Abnormally shaped bones. The space between the head of the humerus and the roof over the joint (the acromion process) is very small. Bone defects or bone abnormalities from a previous injury can make this space even smaller, which can contribute to the problem.

- Muscle weakness and/or joint-capsule stiffness. Weakness in one tissue can cause damage in another. If the joint capsule is tight, for example, the joint cannot function well. The stress caused by a tight joint capsule can lead to impingement, causing pain and weakness.

While ice is a great temporary treatment, the best cure for shoulder impingement is to identify and treat the cause. Consult with a medical professional for a diagnosis. You should also consult with a physical therapist or athletic trainer to answer your questions and address specific issues regarding your child. Specific exercises can strengthen muscles, improve the way the joint works, and stretch tight muscles and tissues.

As a parent or coach, you should decrease pain-causing activities for an athlete with shoulder impingement. Overactivity is the primary cause of this injury for many young athletes. Eager to play, young children often do too much too soon. Decreased activity may mean that your son only throws twenty-five pitches in the baseball game instead of his usual fifty. It may mean your daughter doesn't serve in tennis practice for two days. On the days when injured athletes cannot participate in certain aspects of their sport, they can exercise in other ways to stay in shape. For example, unless your child has dislocated his or her shoulder, running will not hurt it.

Improper technique can lead to shoulder impingement. Identify any flaws in your child's athletic performance. With baseball and softball players, try changing their throwing program or modifying their technique. In other words, if your son plays baseball, you will want to identify any flaws in the way he throws the ball, especially if he pitches. Do the same for your daughter's swimming stroke. If you are unable to evaluate this, contact an athletic trainer, physical therapist, or coach. Simply stopping the activity for a short time without addressing the causes of impingement is only a short-term solution. Once the athlete returns to activity, the problem is likely to reoccur, and it may be even worse than before.

Separated Shoulder

A separated shoulder is another common athletic injury. It is a sprain to the ligaments that support the AC joint, which connects the acromion and the clavicle.

A separated shoulder is usually caused by a direct blow to the shoulder, such as when a hockey player is checked into the boards shoulder first. This sort of injury may involve a bone fracture as well. For this reason, you need to see a physician for x-rays anytime you suspect a shoulder separation.

The degree of separation is often graded from I to III. Grade-I injuries are the least significant and require the least amount of time to heal completely. Grade-III injuries are the most severe and sometimes require surgery.

If the athlete complains of pain at the top of the shoulder, especially where the collarbone meets the acromion, you have a classic sign of shoulder separation. If the child has suffered a shoulder separation, he or she will be unable to move the shoulder very much. Pulling down on the patient's arm will increase the pain.

With a shoulder separation, you may see a deformity. If your child has a severe shoulder separation, ligaments that connect the collarbone to the acromion may rupture. If the ligament ruptures, there is nothing to hold the collarbone down. Therefore, you may see the end of the collarbone stick up an inch or more above the acromion. If you see this, you know your child has a separated shoulder. In serious cases, he or she may need cosmetic surgery.

Always refer shoulder separation injuries to a physician. He or she will take x-rays to rule out fractures and other injuries that also may have occurred. Most of these injuries do not cause nerve damage, as some dislocations do. Calling an ambulance may not be necessary. However, if the athlete displays signs of shock, call 911. Otherwise, transport the child to the doctor as soon as possible.

A shoulder separation can also affect the SC joint. As you recall, the SC joint is the joint where the collarbone attaches to the chest bone. Injuries to this joint are not nearly as common as AC separations, but collision sports (like wrestling) can cause SC joint separations.

SC separations and AC separations have similar symptoms. The difference is in the location of the pain. SC separations hurt in front, where the collarbone attaches to the chest bone. You may also notice a small bump on the chest. This small bump is a good sign, because it indicates an anterior separation (when the collarbone comes in front of the chest bone). This is less serious than a posterior separation.

Posterior separations can be very serious. Because the lungs sit directly behind the SC joint, the collarbone can cause lung damage if it is pushed backward and into the lungs. You may notice a small indentation in the chest if your child has suffered a posterior SC separation. In severe cases, breathing will be difficult, if not labored and painful. Always refer these injuries to a medical professional.

Shoulder Dislocation

When a shoulder becomes dislocated, the humerus comes off the glenoid (it is like the baseball coming off the golf tee). It is intensely painful and limits movement. Although not all dislocations are easy to see with the untrained eye, some look quite grotesque. Sometimes, you will even be able to see the head of the humerus. If you see a deformity, this is a good indication that your child's shoulder is dislocated. In almost all cases, the athlete will have a squared edge to the front or side of his or her shoulder. If possible, compare the injured shoulder with the uninjured one. The healthy shoulder will have a rounded edge.

Shoulder dislocations cause extreme pain and require a trip to the emergency room. You may even wish to call an ambulance. Paramedics are well prepared to treat this injury, especially if the athlete goes into shock. When shoulders dislocate, ligaments, joint capsules, and labral (glenoid labrum) tissues tear. The athlete cannot move the shoulder. The dislocation needs to be treated by a physician as soon as possible. If dislocations occur frequently, the patient may know how to treat it himself or herself; however, we do not recommend this. Nor do we recommend that another person attempt to reduce a shoulder dislocation. If the shoulder isn't "put together" correctly, damage to other tissues (nerves, blood vessels) is possible. In addition, without an x-ray, no one can know if a fracture is involved. Play it safe. Get to a physician immediately.

Once the shoulder has healed, your child might be hesitant to perform the activity that caused the injury. Whether consciously or subconsciously, he or she may limit the joint's range of motion to avoid reinjury. This can cause another set of problems, because it allows the shoulder to become weak. As soon as a doctor clears the athlete for physical activity, encourage the child to get right back in the game.

A primary concern when treating dislocations is to make sure that the injury does not happen again. Athletes under twenty years of age who suffer a traumatic dislocation have a 90 percent chance of reinjury within five years. As the age of the patient increases, the chance of recurrence decreases. However, if you encourage athletes to follow their rehabilitation program diligently, it will help prevent reinjury.

If an athlete's shoulder is dislocated, calm the athlete and be prepared to treat him or her for shock (refer to the Emergency Procedures chapter). Tell the athlete to slow his or her breathing, inhaling through the nose and exhaling slowly through the mouth. Immobilize the arm. If you do not have a sling available, tell the athlete to cradle the injured arm with his or her uninjured arm. Refer the athlete to a physician immediately. You should always call an ambulance if the athlete appears dizzy or lightheaded or if the athlete's fingers lack sensation or blood flow. Do not give the athlete anything to drink before he or she visits the doctor. There are instances in which doctors need to use a general anesthetic to put the shoulder back in place, and drinking beforehand may make the athlete sick.

Physicians will treat a dislocated shoulder with ice and immobilization as soon as possible. Regaining strength and range of motion are an important part of the healing process, but only after the joint has healed. Because each injury is different, your physician will let you know how long you should keep your child's shoulder immobilized. If your child has dislocated his or her shoulder, ask your doctor for a physical therapy order. This guarantees that your child will receive the best instruction and the most appropriate exercises for his or her specific injury.

If your child's shoulder is chronically unstable or if dislocation is the result of a particularly traumatic impact, surgical treatment may be necessary, especially if the dislocation recurs. Following surgery, exercise will help to restore the normal function of the shoulder. Although recovery from shoulder surgery is a lengthy process, most, if not all, athletes bounce back just fine.

Rotator Cuff Tears

Rotator cuff tears can occur in different ways. Acute tears result from a sudden injury, such as when a skier has a high-speed fall.

A chronic tear is the degeneration of the muscle or tendon over time. In the latter case, symptoms may occur either gradually or suddenly. When a tendon is damaged, one minor event may be "the straw that breaks the camel's back." In fact, one patient—a seventy-two-year-old man—went fishing one day. He reached down to pick up a worm and stumbled. He didn't fall to the ground, although he did use his arm to catch himself on a fence. He felt his shoulder pop. He had torn his rotator cuff.

Not all rotator cuff tears are complete. Sometimes the tendon may only be inflamed. Other times, the muscle or tendon fibers may be partially torn, but not completely. Think of the tendon as a rope. As you use the rope, it begins to wear. Over time, you may notice some areas that fray and show signs of wear and tear. Soon, these frayed areas become worse until, eventually, the rope breaks. In this same way, partial rotator cuff tears can become complete tears (also called full-thickness tears) over time.

Pain, weakness, and loss of motion are the most common symptoms of a rotator cuff tear. The pain is usually located in the front of the shoulder joint, just below the acromion process; however, some athletes feel referred pain in the sides of their arm. Patients often cannot raise or lower the arm to their side. If your child displays any of these symptoms, contact your physician.

Fortunately, young athletes do not rupture their rotator cuff very easily. Falling can certainly cause a rotator cuff tear, but this problem is most common in older people. Always ask your doctor or other healthcare provider if you have questions.

Conclusion

Because of its complexity, the shoulder is susceptible to injury. Many baseball, softball, tennis, swimming, and volleyball athletes have experienced shoulder injuries. Athletes in these sports need speed and power to succeed. When a professional baseball player throws a ninety-mile-an-hour fastball, the arm moves from a near standstill to ninety miles an hour in a fraction of a second. Without proper conditioning, this can harm the delicate tissues of the shoulder.

To be good at their sports, athletes need to practice their activities thousands of times. For example, a pitcher could throw 120 pitches in a single game. The athletic trainer at the University of North Carolina once said that his swimmers performed 17,000 strokes per week. The repetitive nature of many of these sports predisposes the shoulder to injury.

Frequently Asked Questions

Q: *My daughter's shoulder hurts when she brushes her hair. Can she still swim?*

A: This is a loaded question. There are two issues here—can she swim, and should she swim. If she has this much pain with daily activities, she likely will not perform as well as she would otherwise. In her case, yes, she can swim. But she should not swim. Swimming in this condition carries more risk as the pain increases. Remember, pain is the body's way of saying, "Hold on! I can't do this anymore!" Consult a physician to identify the cause of your daughter's injury.

Q: *Is heat or ice best?*

A: You will never go wrong with ice. If your daughter ices her shoulder before practice, always make sure that she properly warms up before her practice or event. Sometimes, heat before an event warms up the tissues in preparation for practice or competition. Think of the good rule of thumb: "Heat before; ice after."

Q: *My daughter separated her shoulder in hockey. Will the bump ever go away? Does she need surgery?*

A: These injuries rarely require surgery. Studies show that unless the person requires perfect shoulder anatomy (like a major league baseball pitcher or professional football quarterback), surgery is not necessary—even for serious, Grade-III separations.

However, the bump may be there for a while. Sometimes surgery is the only way to reduce the bump (the elevated collarbone). For cosmetic or aesthetic reasons, this is important to some people.

Q: *My son dislocated his shoulder. Will this happen again?*

A: Most likely, yes. Especially if your son is under twenty years old and participates in contact or overhead sports. Physical therapy, and perhaps surgery, can reduce the chances of recurrence. You will need to ask your physician about this. Doing nothing at all is a great way to ensure another dislocation, however.

Q: *As a "softball mom" and a coach, what can I do to prevent shoulder injuries in my children and players?*

A: Always encourage your children and players to warm up before practice. Never allow anyone to throw hard without proper warm-up. A short game of catch that gradually works into long-distance throwing is great. A light jog—just enough to get a sweat going—will also help.

Encourage your players to seek medical attention if they have shoulder pain. Ignoring shoulder pain only makes the situation worse. Identify the problem as soon as possible.

Follow medical advice. If your son is given specific exercises to do, strongly encourage him to do them. The best athletic trainer or physical therapist in the world can spend every day with your son, but he will not improve unless he does the exercises on his own.

Encourage players to ice after practice. This is especially true at the start of the season and, for pitchers, throughout the season.

Teach proper throwing technique, and be adamant about players throwing correctly. Using the wrong technique can cause injury.

Contributing Author: Mike Muffenbier, MPT, SCS, CSCS

Mike is a physical therapist with the Institute for Athletic Medicine, Braemar Clinic, a clinic that he also supervises. A board-certified clinical specialist, Mike is also coordinator of IAM's Thrower's Injury Program. He teaches rehabilitation professionals throughout the country on the principles of shoulder injury and rehabilitation. Mike and his wife, Michelle, have one daughter, Ali.

Chapter 11

Elbow, Wrist, and Hand Injuries

Baseball and softball players, javelin throwers, and athletes in racquet sports are at risk for elbow pain. However, their symptoms may all be different. One person may have difficulty extending his elbow, while another may have trouble turning the palm of her hand. With wrist or hand pain, your curveball-throwing pitcher can't do nearly as much as he or she can with a healthy hand and wrist.

Anatomy and Biomechanics

Three bones create the elbow joint—the humerus, radius, and ulna. The humerus is the upper arm bone. This bone is part of both the elbow and the shoulder, so it is very important for people in throwing sports. The radius is on the thumb side of the forearm, and it has a rounded portion in the elbow. This rounded portion allows us to turn the palm of our hand down. The ulna is on the pinky side of the forearm, opposite the radius. The ulna forms the point of the elbow.

We can bend and straighten the elbow where the humerus meets the ulna and the radius, and we can turn our palm up and down because of the connection between the radius and the ulna. When the forearm is in its anatomically neutral position, the palm is facing up (you may have noticed this on an anatomical chart). Keep in mind that whenever we refer to the position of the elbow or hand, we will always assume the palm faces up. When the palm faces up, the radius and the ulna are almost parallel. When the palm faces down, the radius has crossed over the ulna. All this motion comes from the elbow.

The muscles on the outside of the elbow on the thumb side extend the wrist (bending the palm backward), while the muscles on the inside of the elbow flex the wrist (bending the palm forward). Forearm muscles also control specific movement in the hand and wrist. Overuse injuries are common in the forearm and elbow.

Several muscles control specific finger and hand movements. These muscles travel down the forearm from the elbow and into the wrist. At the wrist, they turn into tendons and are housed in small, tunnel-like compartments.

Ligaments connect the bones of the elbow. The medial collateral ligament connects the ulna to the humerus (the upper arm bone). The lateral collateral ligament connects the radius to the humerus. Both ligaments provide stability to the joint. Sprains to the elbow are not uncommon. Sports like football, hockey, wrestling, and gymnastics place a great deal of stress on these ligaments, so elbow injuries are common in these sports. However, overuse and repetition in noncontact sports can cause injury to these ligaments as well.

Many small bones—the carpals, the metacarpals, and the phalanges—make up the wrist and hand. The ulna and the radius meet these smaller bones to make up the wrist. The carpals bones form two rows of four bones inside the wrist (eight bones total). The row closest to the forearm lies on top of the radius and ulna. A cartilage called the triangular fibrocartilage provides support on the ulnar side of the wrist and separates the ulna from the carpal bones. Ligaments (twenty-one of them in the wrist) and tendons connect these bones, providing stability to the joints.

Metacarpal bones form the hand, and they meet with the carpal bones near the wrist. Physicians and other medical providers refer to these bones by numbers: the first metacarpal connects the thumb, the second connects the index finger, and so on. Again, ligaments connect these bones together, and tendons connect these bones to muscles. This is what allows us to squeeze objects, such as a baseball or softball. Forceful contact with an opponent or an immovable object (punching a wall, for example) can fracture these bones.

Left Hand (viewed from the palm)

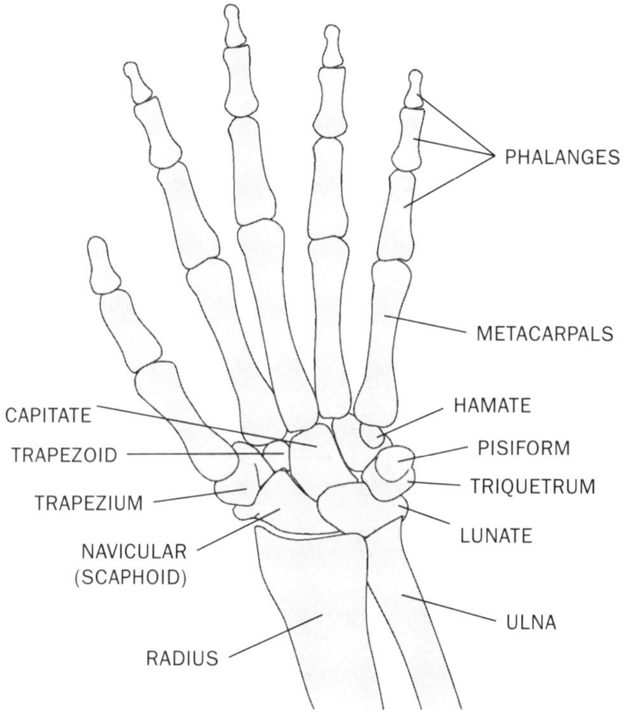

LifeART Collection Images © 1989-1997 TechPool Studios, Inc. USA

The phalanges are the small bones that make up our fingers. We refer to the joints that form between the phalanges as knuckles. Often, we see fractures and dislocations of these bones. Even more often, we see sprains and inflammation of the ligaments that connect these bones and the tendons that control finger movement. This latter type of injury can sometimes be classified as a "jammed finger."

Elbow Injuries

Epicondylitis

Medial epicondylitis and lateral epicondylitis are very similar injuries. Both are injuries to the muscles and tendons that attach at the elbow and control certain wrist and hand activities. Medial epicondylitis occurs on the inside of the elbow (the pinky side). Some people call this "little league elbow." Lateral epicondylitis occurs on the outside of the elbow (the thumb side), and is often referred to as "tennis elbow." Tennis elbow is three to four times more common than little league elbow, and it affects more than just tennis players. Carpenters and electricians often have lateral epicondylitis because they constantly use their elbows at work (to turn screws, for example).

These elbow injuries hurt, especially during activity. The location of the pain depends on the injury. Little league elbow causes pain on the inside of the elbow where the muscles meet near the elbow joint. With this injury, activities as simple as curling the wrist or throwing a ball are both difficult and painful. Tennis elbow, on the other hand, causes pain on the outside of the elbow where the muscles meet the elbow joint. With this injury, movements such as a backhand in tennis or the use of a motorcycle throttle cause pain. Patients with medial or lateral epicondylitis sometimes say that the pain radiates down the arm and can last from one to three days after activity. For most people, the pain is gradual and causes the most problems during and immediately following activity.

If your daughter has little league elbow, she will have weakness when she tries to curl her wrist upward while you push it downward, resisting her motion. Your tennis-playing son may have weakness with activities that involve wrist extension (the same motion as using the throttle on a motorcycle). Weakness can translate into decreased performance. Watch your child perform. You may notice that the child doesn't throw the softball quite as hard or serve as forcefully in tennis as he or she used to. This could indicate injury.

Both of these injuries are treated in a similar manner. RICE will reduce pain and inflammation, but keep in mind that relative rest means avoiding activities that cause pain. Baseball players should avoid throwing, and tennis players should avoid playing tennis. Your child may do other activities, however, such as quickness and agility drills and other cardiovascular exercises.

Strengthening exercises, like wrist curls and wrist extensions, are good therapy as well. Because it is important to work on muscle balance throughout recovery, we always tell people to strengthen the entire joint, even if one muscle group doesn't hurt. Elbow flexion and extension exercises are good for these injuries, too. A physician, physical therapist, or athletic trainer can recommend specific stretches and exercises for your child.

Your doctor may recommend an over-the-counter medication like Ibuprofen. This works well to reduce inflammation and control pain. If you have further questions, ask your doctor or pharmacist.

Ligament Sprains

Earlier, we mentioned that the bones in the elbow are connected by ligaments. The medial collateral ligament connects the ulna to the humerus (the upper arm bone). The lateral collateral ligament connects the radius to the humerus. Both ligaments provide stability to the joint. Either acute or chronic injuries can damage these ligaments. An acute injury, such as a hyperextension or dislocation, occurs quite suddenly, whereas a chronic injury is an injury that gradually worsens over time.

Injuries to these ligaments cause specific pain, and athletes can usually point to the spot that hurts the most. Localized swelling also is quite common. Athletes usually feel pain during an activity, and the pain may increase considerably afterward. Lateral collateral ligament injuries hurt on the outside of the elbow; medial collateral ligament injuries hurt on the inside of the elbow. Because ligaments connect bone to bone, ligament injuries can make joints feel loose or less stable. Pain and instability can cause loss of strength. Watch your child perform—you may be surprised at how much information you can get about an injury simply by watching.

You probably noticed that the symptoms for ligament sprains look a lot like those for epicondylitis injuries. For this reason, physicians, athletic trainers, and physical therapists often have trouble determining the extent of an elbow injury. Physicians will often order an MRI and other diagnostic tests to confirm the nature of an injury.

Treatment of ligament injuries is similar to the treatment of epicondylitis. RICE and anti-inflammatory medication help treat the initial symptoms. Stretching and strengthening exercises help stabilize the joint and prevent further injury. You may want to invest in an elbow brace to provide added stability. You may also want to ask a physical therapist or an athletic trainer for recommendations about specific elbow braces.

Bursitis

Remember how the tip of Popeye's elbow stuck out? This is what people with olecranon bursitis (inflammation to the bursa sac) have: "Popeye Elbow."

The olecranon process is the portion of your ulna (the forearm bone on the pinky side) that creates the bony point at the tip of your elbow. The olecranon bursa, then, is the bursa sac (a fluid-filled sac providing shock absorption and reducing friction) that sits near or on the olecranon process. Because it is very close to the skin, it doesn't have a lot of protection, so it becomes infected more easily than other bursae in the body.

Olecranon bursitis can happen because of an acute or traumatic episode, like falling on your elbow in hockey, or it can happen as a chronic, overuse injury. It often looks worse than it really is. Patients usually have a big, fluid-filled "sac" on the tip of their elbow. Olecranon bursitis usually doesn't cause a lot of pain (ligament, tendon, and bone injuries, on the other hand, can cause a lot of pain). When you touch the injury, it feels spongy, like water in a balloon.

A high-school hockey player fell on his elbow during playoffs. The injured elbow became swollen, but it wasn't very painful, so he didn't mention it to anybody. His elbow remained sore, but he managed to do everything he wanted to do. When he started baseball practice in the spring, he noticed that the elbow was still swollen. Then, one day, he dove for a ball and landed on the tip of his elbow. Within minutes, the elbow looked ten times its normal size. Although he had first injured his bursa sac during hockey, his second injury aggravated the problem, causing the bursitis.

With bursitis, physicians usually prefer to help the body's natural healing process through RICE and anti-inflammatory medication. However, in some cases, particularly the lingering cases, a physician may elect to drain the bursa. In one case, the athlete's physician opted to drain the bursa sac because it was a chronic condition and excessively swollen. The athlete took three days off and did not have elbow pain for the rest of the season.

Keep in mind that despite their ghoulish appearance, not all bursa injuries are serious. Ice these injuries as often as possible and wrap the injury with an ACE bandage. This provides compression and limits the extent of the swelling.

Ulnar Nerve Injury

When your daughter says she hit her "funny bone," she really is saying that she injured her ulnar nerve. In most cases, this pain lasts only a few seconds, and there may be some slight tingling into the fingers. Because the nerve is close to the surface of the skin, it is predisposed to injury. Most people do not experience lingering problems; however, if the injury does not resolve within a few minutes, contact your physician or emergency facility.

Weight lifters, hockey players, racquet sport players, and athletes involved in throwing sports will occasionally suffer ulnar nerve injuries. In some cases, these injuries can cause significant discomfort and loss of motor function. Some athletes will describe this sensation as a heavy or clumsy hand.

If an ulnar nerve injury is chronic or repeated, we recommend a visit to the physician. There are several causes for these chronic cases. Sometimes, the nerve can slip out of its groove (the tunnel through which the nerve runs). It can also become entrapped in the groove. Much of the time, patients are prone to injury because they have inherited a groove that is narrow or irregular. Bone spurs in the groove can also irritate the nerve.

Remember that nerves carry information to our muscles. Nerve impulses allow muscles to contract, which allows us to grasp things and perform motor activities like eating and buttoning our shirts. Long-term problems with the ulnar nerve can affect more than just athletic performance.

Elbow Fractures and Dislocations

Elbow fractures are almost always acute injuries. Some athletes experience stress fractures, but complete elbow fractures are usually the result of trauma. Examples of traumatic injuries are falling out of a tree, landing on the elbow after being tackled, or slipping on the pool deck. Given their inquisitive and competitive nature, children are at particular risk for these types of injuries.

It is also possible to dislocate the elbow. A dislocation occurs when an acute injury displaces the radius or ulna. This injury will tear ligaments and sometimes tendons as well. If the child is unable to bend the elbow, and you notice a deformity, splint and immobilize the elbow, treat for shock, and take the child to the emergency room.

Look for the following symptoms:

- Pain. Like all fractures, these injuries hurt. Touch the three bones of the elbow. One or all may be painful.
- Deformities. Touch the elbow to feel for deformity. You may need to compare the injured side with the uninjured side.
- Extreme swelling and discoloration. Note, however, that while these are common responses to fractures, they could indicate another type of injury as well.

If you suspect that your child has an elbow fracture, immobilize the joint and contact your doctor's office. X-rays are the only way to be certain of an elbow fracture.

Forearm Fractures

Broken arms are common, especially in curious young children. These injuries are often easy to detect. Like other fractures, they cause intense pain and swelling, and grip strength is usually much weaker on the broken arm than on the uninjured arm.

Because the forearm bones are so prominent, deformities are usually easy to detect. If you see a bump in the middle of your daughter's arm, chances are that the arm is broken. Immobilize the arm and bring your child to the doctor. In most cases, six to eight weeks in a cast is all that is needed to heal the arm.

Wrist and Hand Injuries

Sprains

Sprains are one of the most common injuries to the wrist. They usually occur when an athlete falls on a hyperextended wrist, which happens quite often in athletic activity. Forced wrist flexion can also cause injuries to the ligaments and bones, but this occurs less frequently. As common as wrist and hand injuries are, they are often mismanaged.

Like other sprains that may occur throughout the body, a wrist sprain causes pain, a burning sensation, and weakness. As you may recall, tendonitis also may cause pain, a burning sensation, and weakness. However, unlike tendonitis, wrist sprains sometimes produce audible "pops" or "snaps," which may indicate that more structural damage was done.

To care for a wrist sprain, first rule out a fracture. Check the athlete's grip strength. Good grip strength and motion suggests a sprain, not a fracture. For severe sprains (sprains that significantly limit wrist motion or cause a lot of pain, clicking, or popping), athletes should see a physician for an x-ray.

Next, ice the injury to reduce inflammation and control swelling. Then, wrap the wrist lightly with an ACE bandage to provide support and help control swelling. Later, it is likely that a hand therapist will make a splint to immobilize the joint for several weeks. When your young athlete can tolerate it, have him or her start squeezing a soft sponge or Silly-Putty. The hand therapist can answer any questions you may have and guide your child through rehabilitation.

Fractures

Wrist fractures are possible, especially to the ends of the radius and ulna. A wrist fracture hurts like crazy, and your child will likely see a deformity. These injuries (sometimes called Colles fracture, Smith's fracture, or Barton's fracture) can be serious. If not treated properly, they can damage blood vessels, nerves, and growth plates. Therefore, always refer wrist fractures to an urgent care or emergency room immediately.

Depending on the severity of the fracture, surgery may or may not be necessary. With or without surgery, physicians typically cast wrist fractures for six to eight weeks. Encourage your child to practice range-of-motion exercises on the noncasted areas to prevent stiffness. Recovery times vary, but stiff fingers and hand muscles prolong recovery. As always, your child should see an athletic trainer or hand therapist for strengthening exercises after these injuries.

The scaphoid bone (also called the navicular bone) is located at the base of the thumb. It is the most frequently injured carpal bone, which sits in an area called the "anatomical snuffbox." To find this area, spread your thumb and fingers apart as far as they can and lift up your thumb. You should notice two very prominent tendons at the base of your thumb. The anatomical snuffbox is between these two tendons.

Scaphoid injury usually occurs when an athlete falls on his or her outstretched arm and lands on the hand with the wrist bent backward. The more the wrist is bent, the greater the odds of fracturing the scaphoid. This bone is unique, because it does not have a good blood supply. For this reason, scaphoid injuries take a long time to heal.

With a scaphoid injury, the athlete will have pain or point tenderness on the bone and may suffer persistent swelling on the back and thumb side of the wrist. Wrist movement and grip strength (squeezing someone's hand) will be painful.

If you suspect a fracture, immobilize and RICE the wrist, then contact your physician. Even your physician may not know right away if your child has fractured the scaphoid. Often, the first x-ray will not show a scaphoid fracture. Your doctor may need two or even three different sets of x-rays (each two to three weeks apart) to determine the nature of the injury. If your child's wrist does not improve—even after negative x-rays—your doctor may order a bone scan.

The scaphoid takes a long time to heal. Treatment options include a cast, surgery, and/or therapy. Your child may need as much as twelve to thirty weeks in a cast for the bone to heal properly. If, after casting, the scaphoid still has not healed properly, a surgeon may need to place a screw or pin into the scaphoid. Again, recovery time varies, but patients usually wear a cast for four weeks after the surgery and can begin light active motion after that. After either immobilization or surgery, you should contact a hand therapist for rehabilitation. In most cases, athletes will continue to have wrist stiffness, even with therapy. Recovery from a scaphoid injury can be a lengthy process. Try to prepare your child for the long haul.

Another common carpal fracture is to the hamate bone. In most cases, this involves a small portion (called the "hook") of the hamate that extends into the palm. The fracture usually happens from a direct fall onto the bone, or from the force of an uncontrolled bat, racquet, or club that strikes the bone. If your child has fractured the hamate, he or she may have tenderness and swelling over the muscular pad on the palm side of the pinky, pain while bending the pinky finger (especially flexion), a weak and painful grip, and/or numbness in the pinky. Depending on the severity of the break, a physician will likely cast the fracture for six to twelve weeks. If it does not heal properly, your physician may elect to remove the hook of the hamate.

Falls and collisions in contact sports can cause wrist fractures. Certainly, any one of the eight bones in the wrist may break, and the symptoms will be similar to those we have highlighted. Always contact your physician if you suspect a fracture.

Tendonitis

To the untrained eye, tendonitis may resemble a sprain. Both injuries can cause pain, a burning sensation, and weakness. However, unlike sprains (which result from acute, traumatic injury), tendonitis occurs when the muscles and/or tendons are used with too much repetition. It can also occur if ligaments fail to support the carpal bones. (If an athlete sprains his or her wrist, for example, his or her muscles and tendons must work overtime to stabilize the wrist.) Both cases cause inflammation and pain.

Suspect tendonitis if your child experiences prolonged aching or burning, especially with activity. This is gradual pain that worsens over time. Be concerned about pain—especially intense pain—that gets worse over just two or three weeks. With tendonitis, the pain decreases when your child is inactive.

Carpal Tunnel Syndrome

Carpal tunnel syndrome is a common injury these days. This injury is caused by compression of the median nerve as it travels through the tunnels in the wrist. Many people—secretaries, butchers, factory workers, and even athletes—have carpal tunnel syndrome. What do these people have in common? They are all likely to use their wrists repetitively. But not all wrist pain is related to carpal tunnel syndrome.

Carpal tunnel syndrome has several defining characteristics. Sufferers may experience persistent tingling and numbness on the palm side of the thumb, index finger, middle finger, and/or ring finger, with or without activity. Other symptoms include weakness, poor motor control, loss of muscle mass on the palm of the hand, and shooting pain that radiates from the hand or wrist into the forearm. If the nerve becomes compressed, it may lose the ability to communicate with other muscles and tissues. When this happens, patients inexplicably drop things and lose the ability to perform simple, routine tasks.

If you suspect that your child has carpal tunnel syndrome, contact a physician immediately. Your physician will likely order that your child stop the activity that causes pain. He or she may also order a splint and anti-inflammatory medication.

Ganglion Cyst

A ganglion cyst is a fluid-filled lump that can appear anywhere on the wrist, but usually appears on the back side. This cyst or lump usually comes from within the wrist joint. Most ganglion cysts are painless, although some will cause pain at first. Ganglion cysts may cause pain when they grow, and they might interfere with the structures around them. These cysts are almost always benign and do not interfere with performance.

Treatment for these cysts varies. Your physician may elect to drain the cyst with a needle or make a tiny incision and remove the lump. If you think your child may have a ganglion cyst, don't worry. As long as the cyst isn't painful, it may not be crucial to see a physician immediately. Make an appointment with your doctor to rule out any serious conditions.

Finger Injuries

Many of us have injured our fingers playing sports. Basketball players, especially, know what this is like. However, not every injury is a simple jammed finger. In fact, some injuries can lead to permanent deformity if left untreated.

Mallet Finger

Mallet finger is common in basketball and baseball. This injury occurs when a ball strikes the tip of the finger, causing one of the tendons to rupture or avulse (see page 130). These injuries hurt, and athletes will be unable to fully straighten the tip of their finger. Ice and splint the finger so it is totally straight before going to the doctor for x-rays. (Popsicle sticks work great as finger splints.)

Boutonniere Deformity

Boutonniere deformity is another tendon injury. In this case, the tendon ruptures in the top part of the middle of the finger. Athletes with this injury are unable to straighten the top half of their finger. Obviously, this injury also hurts. Ice it, splint it, keep it straight, and take your child to the doctor.

Jersey Finger

Jersey finger is another tendon injury. Unlike the previous two injuries, however, the injured tendon in this case comes off the palm side of the finger, making it difficult for the athlete to bend the fingertip. If the athlete cannot bend the last joint on his or her finger, this is a red flag indicating that the athlete should see a doctor right away. Jersey finger can be serious, because it may cause people to lose the ability to pinch objects and perform other daily tasks we take for granted.

Unfortunately, surgical repair is necessary with jersey finger. Because people often mistake this injury for a sprain, you should ask a physician to evaluate all finger injuries to ensure proper treatment.

Gamekeeper's Thumb

Gamekeeper's thumb is a ligament injury that occurs when the thumb is twisted or when an athlete falls on his or her outstretched thumb. Skiers and football players are particularly at risk for this injury. With gamekeeper's thumb, the ligament on the inside of the thumb (where the thumb meets the rest of the hand) tears, either partially or completely. Pain, swelling, and some discoloration will occur. Because this ligament provides a lot of stability for the thumb, this injury can be serious.

Surgical repair may or may not be necessary. Some athletes get better using only a splint. If your child plays quarterback, however, the stability of the thumb is much more important than if your child runs track and field, so surgery may be the more appropriate treatment. Steve played quarterback for his high-school football team. He suffered gamekeeper's thumb, but he did not have his thumb surgically repaired. His grip strength and the accuracy of his passes suffered. In retrospect, he should have had the surgery.

If you suspect a thumb sprain, ice the injury, then lightly wrap the thumb with an ACE bandage for support and comfort. If the injury doesn't improve within a few days, see your physician.

Sprains

Finger sprains are the typical jammed fingers that we hear so much about. Just like the knee and the elbow, the finger has collateral ligaments that connect the joints. These ligaments can be injured just like any other ligaments in the body.

Finger sprains hurt, and some even appear fractured. Swelling often persists for a couple of weeks. Most finger sprains happen because of a force to the end of the finger, like when a volleyball or basketball strikes the fingertip. The pain is located near the joint, especially on the sides (where the ligaments are). The joint is unstable when tested by a medical professional.

Ice and immobilize these injuries right away. Athletic tape may be an acceptable substitute for splinting, as long as the joint shows no other signs of fracture. Never pull on a jammed finger—this may cause additional damage. If the injury doesn't improve within a few days, see a doctor for x-rays.

Fractures

With finger fractures, grip strength suffers, and patients can't squeeze anything without feeling a lot of pain. If you look closely enough, you may also see a deformity. Keep in mind that if there is enough force to fracture a bone, there may be enough force to tear ligaments and other supporting tissues as well.

Treat this injury the same way you would treat a sprain: Ice and immobilize the finger until you can get x-rays. Not all fractured fingers require a trip to the emergency room. If your son injures his finger late Friday night during a football game, consider waiting until the morning to see your physician—unless, of course, the finger is deformed or the fracture causes uncontrollable pain. You can manage the injury at home by keeping it taped or splinted, icing the injury every hour or two, and providing pain medication, such as Tylenol, as needed.

Your child will need x-rays; however, other patients may take priority over a finger injury in the emergency room. This means that you could wait up to several hours for treatment. It may be more beneficial for your child to rest until the morning. Make an appointment at your physician's office the next day.

Dislocations

Finger dislocations occur when the ligaments and other supporting tissues tear, causing the bones to "come out of place." As with sprains and fractures, this can happen when a ball strikes the end of the finger (like in basketball or volleyball). Because dislocated fingers are so deformed, they are difficult to miss. Even the untrained eye can spot a finger dislocation.

While finger dislocations are easy to reduce (put back in place), we do not recommend that you try it. Ice and immobilize these injuries and go to the physician right away.

Conclusion

We have only scratched the surface with these elbow, wrist, hand, and finger injuries. These injuries are difficult for even trained professionals to manage, so we don't expect you to become an expert in the field. However, we do want you to think about some of the more serious injuries and recognize injuries that could cause deformity.

Elbow injuries affect many athletes, especially those who play softball and baseball. Because the muscles that control hand, wrist, and finger motion start at the elbow, elbow injures can affect other activities involving the hand or wrist.

Hand and finger injuries are common in athletics as well. When evaluating these injuries, compare the injured side of the body to the unaffected side. Pay special attention to deformities. Always see a doctor for finger injuries, especially if pain persists. Some may require immediate treatment.

Finally, pay special attention to grip strength, which can tell you a great deal about an injury's severity. John, a soccer goalie, had his hand stepped on during a game. The next day, the athletic trainer examined his swollen, discolored hand. On the surface, the hand looked as if it may have been fractured. However, his grip strength was perfect. Hand fractures, which cause considerable pain, greatly reduce grip strength. John's injury was simply a bruise.

Frequently Asked Questions

Q: *My daughter jammed her finger. It is swollen. Should we be worried?*

A: You have reason to be concerned. If the finger appears normal (no deformities, fully straight), you can afford to be patient. Ice the injury and work on range of motion. "Buddy tape" the finger for competitions (tape the injured finger to the uninjured finger next to it, above and below the joint). Seek assistance after three to four days if the finger does not improve at all.

If the finger doesn't fully straighten, especially at the tip, see your doctor right away. Your daughter could have mallet finger, which is an injury that often results in an avulsion fracture or ruptured tendon. She may or may not need surgery to correct this problem, but your doctor should make that decision.

Q: *Is it okay for my son to throw curveballs? He is only ten years old.*

A: Little league elbow, also called medial epicondylitis, can possibly result from throwing too many curveballs with poor technique.

We typically don't recommend that young children throw curveballs until they reach thirteen or fourteen years old. We say this for two reasons. First, their muscles aren't yet strong enough to withstand the stresses of throwing a curveball. Second, most young children can't throw the curveball for strikes anyway. They end up walking too many batters when they throw the curve. Tell your son to stick with the fastball and to work on his pinpoint control.

Q: *My son said his fingers tingle when he plays football, especially when he is tackled. Any suggestions?*

A: There are many possible causes for this. One is a direct blow to the ulnar nerve—the "funny bone." These injuries last only a few seconds and usually resolve without any medical attention. If your son's fingers tingle after he is struck in the elbow, chances are good that he hit his "funny bone." Another potential cause is carpal tunnel, although this injury is generally a result of repetitive activity, not contact in football. Another possibility is that the tingling could be referred pain from your son's neck. Cervical disc injuries can produce this same symptom. You should contact a healthcare provider for this one.

Q: *Is cracking your knuckles bad for you? I have heard it causes arthritis.*

A: Probably not. Most experts agree that cracking your knuckles does not cause arthritis. The sound you hear is the gases escaping from within the joint. It does not cause arthritis. Aunt Mabel may have arthritis—and she may have cracked her knuckles—but she most likely developed arthritis from something else.

Contributing Author: James Buesgens, OTR

James is an Occupational Therapist with Fairview Hand Center in Edina, Minnesota. A 1992 Honors Graduate of Creighton University, James specializes in hand therapy and currently lectures resident orthopedic surgeons on topics in hand therapy. James, a member of the American Society of Hand Therapists, lives in Lonsdale, Minnesota.

Contributing Author: Scott Kulstad, MEd, ATC/R

Questions for Your Doctor

You have the right to ask your physician any questions that will affect your child's care. If your child needs medical attention, please keep the following questions in mind.

1. *Does my child need x-rays?*
2. *When can my child return to full competition?*
3. *How long and how often does he or she have to wear this splint/brace?*
4. *What will the outcome of this treatment be?*
5. *What can cause reinjury and how do we prevent it?*
6. *How much pain should the child experience with this injury?*
7. *What can I do to help control my child's pain?*
8. *Will he or she have limitations from this injury?*
9. *If surgery is necessary, what would the surgery involve?*
10. *Will therapy assist in a better outcome for this injury?*
11. *What are the risks in playing with this injury?*
12. *How long will rehabilitation take?*

Suggested Readings

American Medical Association Pocket Guide to Sports First Aid. New York: Random House, 1996.

Andrews, James R., and William G. Clancy, Jr., eds. *On-Field Evaluation and Treatment of Common Athletic Injuries.* St. Louis, Mo.: Mosby-Year Book, 1997.

Ellis, Joe, and Joe Henderson. *Running Injury-Free: How to Prevent, Treat and Recover from Dozens of Painful Problems.* Emmaus, Pa.: Rodale Press, 1994.

Griffith, H. Winter. *Complete Guide to Sports Injuries: How to Treat Fractures, Bruises, Sprains, Strains, Dislocations, Head Injuries.* New York: Perigee, 1997.

Michel, Lyle J., and Mark Jenkins. *The Sports Medicine Bible: Prevent, Detect, and Treat Your Sports Injuries through the Latest Medical Techniques.* New York: HarperCollins, 1995.

Peterson, Marilyn S. *Eat to Compete: A Guide to Sports Nutrition.* St. Louis, Mo.: Mosby-Year Book, 1996.

Potparic, O., and J. Gibson. *A Dictionary of Sports Injuries and Disorders.* Pearl River, N.Y.: Parthenon Pub. Group, 1996.

Reider, Bruce, ed. *Sports Medicine: The School Age Athlete.* Philadelphia: W.B. Saunders, 1996.

Taylor, William N. *Anabolic Steroids and the Athlete.* Jefferson, N.C.: McFarland & Co., 1982.

Online Resources

American Dietetic Association
http://www.eatright.org

American Medical Association
http://www.ama-assn.org

American Orthopedic Society for Sports Medicine: Ask the Sports Doctor
http://www.sportsmed.org/d/d.htm

American Physical Therapy Association
www.apta.org

Coaches and Athletic Trainers Corner
http://www.clark.net/pub/aapsm/coachindex.html

Institute for Athletic Medicine—Fairview Health Services
www.Fairview.org/iam

Mayo Clinic Health Oasis: Daily News on Disease, Treatment, Drugs, Diet
http://www.mayohealth.org

Minnesota Athletic Trainers' Association
www.glata.org/minnesota

The National Athletic Trainers' Association
www.nata.org

The Physician and Sports Medicine Online
http://www.physsportsmed.com

Index